Advances in Kidney Transplantation

Edited by Rafael Fernández Castillo

Published in London, United Kingdom

Advances in Kidney Transplantation
http://dx.doi.org/10.5772/intechopen.1003483
Edited by Rafael Fernández Castillo

Contributors
Aida Hamzić-Mehmedbašić, Alison Vannia Nava Rojas, Arry Rodjani, Azra Ribić-Mrkonja, Damir Rebić, David Andrés Ballesteros Castro, Diana Vetter, Ernest Kwame Adjepong-Tandoh, Gede Wirya Kusuma Duarsa, Gerhard Reinaldi Situmorang, Israel Danny Rivas Salazar, Karen Courville, Maiko Alejandro Tavera Díaz, Merima Odobašić, Mohammad Hassan Al-thnaibat, Norman Bustamante, Nur Rasyid, Omar Lafuente Covarrubias, Pande Made Wisnu Tirtayasa, Thomas Schachtner, Vedad Herenda

First published in London, United Kingdom, 2025 by IntechOpen
IntechOpen is the global imprint of INTECHOPEN LIMITED, registered in England and Wales, registration number: 11086078, 167-169 Great Portland Street, London, W1W 5PF, United Kingdom

For EU product safety concerns: IN TECH d.o.o., Prolaz Marije Krucifikse Kozulić 3, 51000 Rijeka, Croatia, info@intechopen.com or visit our website at intechopen.com.

British Library Cataloguing-in-Publication Data
A catalogue record for this book is available from the British Library

Advances in Kidney Transplantation
Edited by Rafael Fernández Castillo
p. cm.
Print ISBN 978-1-83769-964-3
Online ISBN 978-1-83769-963-6
eBook (PDF) ISBN 978-1-83769-965-0

Meet the editor

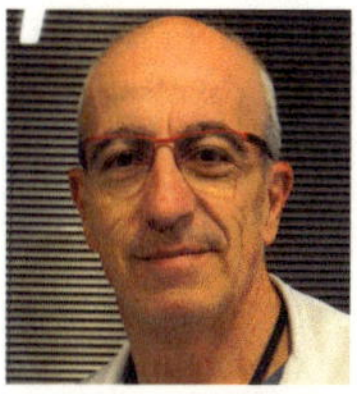

Rafael Fernández Castillo is a renowned researcher with extensive experience in the field of nephrology and renal transplantation. He has been the principal investigator in various projects on immunosuppression, immunological compatibility, and postoperative management in transplant patients. His approach combines clinical excellence with a strong academic track record, publishing numerous articles in high-impact scientific journals. He is currently a full professor at a prestigious university and leads a multidisciplinary team dedicated to innovation in advanced renal therapies. His commitment to training new generations of specialists and his participation in international conferences have established him as a prominent figure in his field.

Contents

Preface

It is both an honour and a privilege to present this volume entitled *Advances in Kidney Transplantation*, a book that brings together the contributions of renowned experts in a field as fundamental and transformative as this within modern medicine. Throughout its chapters, readers will find a deep and comprehensive insight into the most recent advances in kidney transplantation, a subject that not only represents a technical and scientific achievement but also reflects the ethical and human commitment to improving the quality of life of those suffering from chronic kidney disease.

Kidney transplantation has evolved significantly since its inception, establishing itself as the best therapeutic option for patients with end-stage renal disease. However, this medical practice continues to face considerable challenges, ranging from the scarcity of available organs and the difficulties of immunosuppression to the need for personalised treatments that address the diversity of clinical cases. This volume tackles these challenges from multiple perspectives, integrating the latest knowledge in biology, surgery, pharmacology, ethics, and health policies.

The selection of topics included in this book reflects both the richness and complexity of kidney transplantation. Among these, we highlight advances in surgical techniques, the development of new, less toxic immunosuppressive strategies, and research into biomarkers that enable more precise detection of acute or chronic rejection. Additionally, fundamental aspects such as initiatives to increase organ availability through live donation programmes and transplants with marginal donors are explored. These issues are becoming increasingly relevant in the context of growing global demand.

Beyond the technical aspects, this book also delves into the ethical and social issues underlying kidney transplantation. Inequities in access to treatment, differences between healthcare systems in various countries, and decisions regarding patient prioritisation on waiting lists are among the topics that invite us to reflect on how to ensure that scientific advances go hand in hand with social justice.

I want to express my deepest gratitude to the authors who have contributed their time and expertise to bring this work to life. Each chapter reflects the effort and dedication of experts passionate about their field, whose commitment to research and clinical practice enables continuous progress in this vital area. This book would not have been possible without their generous willingness to share their knowledge and experiences.

Furthermore, I would like to highlight the essential role of the editorial team in this project. Their tireless collaboration, expertise in the field, and attention to detail have been key factors in the quality and coherence of this volume. Their work has enabled the creation of a book that we hope will become a valuable resource for health professionals, researchers, students, and all those interested in kidney transplantation.

Finally, I want to extend my gratitude to the patients and their families, who are not only the raison d'être of this collective effort but also a constant source of inspiration. Their courage, resilience, and trust in science and medical professionals remind us daily of the importance of our work.

I sincerely hope that this volume provides valuable and up-to-date information, inspires new ideas, fosters interdisciplinary collaboration, and contributes to advancing this crucial field. Beyond being an academic text, this work seeks to be a meeting point for reflection, innovation, and, above all, continued efforts to transform lives through kidney transplantation.

Rafael Fernández Castillo
University of Granada,
Biosanitary Research Institute,
Granada, Spain

Section 1

Updates on Chronic Kidney Disease

Chapter 1

Advancing Kidney Transplantation in Developing Countries

Ernest Kwame Adjepong-Tandoh

Abstract

Chronic kidney disease (CKD) and end-stage renal disease (ESRD) in developing countries are characterized by increasing prevalence and incidence rates. Provision of renal replacement therapy has not kept pace with the ever-growing burden of disease, leading to limited accessibility and poor patient outcomes. Advancing kidney transplantation (KT) in these regions is fraught with major challenges such as poverty and limited financial commitment, shortage of appropriate infrastructure and logistics, inadequate trained professionals, and limited donor pool. Absence of required legislature on organ donation and regulatory oversights retard the establishment, progress, and sustainability of transplant programmes. Despite these hurdles, significant progress has been chalked in some regions through innovative approaches and strategic interventions. This chapter evaluates the key barriers to KT in developing countries and offers insights and strategies from successful models in other countries. Some recommendations include expanding existing infrastructure, exploring effective training options for health professionals, and fostering international and private partners collaborations. Through these efforts, developing countries can improve access to KT and ultimately enhance the lives of patients with ESRD.

Keywords: kidney transplantation, end stage renal disease, chronic kidney disease, developing countries, renal replacement therapy

1. Introduction

Kidney diseases are a major global health concern that have a substantial impact on both individuals and healthcare systems worldwide. The burden of kidney disease is still disproportionately high in developing countries, where resources and healthcare infrastructure are often limited, despite advances in medical technology and treatments. Epidemiological data reveal stark contrasts between developed and developing countries in terms of the prevalence and incidence rates of chronic kidney disease (CKD) and end-stage renal disease (ESRD).

Of the global prevalence of 500 million people (8 to 16%) affected by CKD and estimate of 78% (387.5 million) are in low-income to middle-income countries [1, 2], a large proportion of which lack access to kidney disease prevention, diagnosis, or treatment [3].

2. Economic and social impact of kidney disease

Managing CKD and dialysis can consume up to 3% of the national healthcare budget in developed countries, despite representing a small fraction of the population. In developing countries, however, the financial burden often falls on patients and their families due to limited health insurance coverage and/or government funding.

The high cost of treatment can cause untold economic hardships for patients and their supporting families. Beyond the direct healthcare expenses incurred by the affected patient, CKD results in significant productivity losses. The negative effects on the overall national productivity and economic growth are often underappreciated but important. More concerning is that most CKD patients in developing countries are in their productive years [1, 4–33], a sharp contrast to the older age groups in the developed world [34], further worsening the economic impact.

Patients with CKD suffer significant social impairment from the symptoms of the disease and the side effects of the treatment, with the potential of disrupting their family and social lives. The relative lack of mental healthcare services in developing countries leads to inadequate treatment of CKD-related mental issues like anxiety and depression are not adequately addressed.

Approximately 93% of the world's population on receiving renal replacement therapy(RRT) lives in high-income countries (HICs) or upper-middle-income countries, which comprise only 52% of the world population [35, 36]. Successful kidney transplantation (KT) has been achievable for over 50 years, and in developed countries, it has evolved from an experimental procedure to a standard option in RRT. Progress in KT has been in tandem with advancements in dialysis, resulting in a situation where virtually everyone who develops ESRD in these countries receives either dialysis or KT. Consequently, very few patients die due to a lack of treatment [37].

Unfortunately, an often-contrasting situation is observed in developing countries. Here, only a minority of patients progressing to ESRD receive adequate RRT [37, 38], and the number receiving KT is small and unevenly distributed. Since RRT is expensive and its benefit is not adequately quantified in developing economies, its development has understandably lagged behind efforts toward tackling infectious diseases and other healthcare burdens [37]. However, the limited attention and resource allocation to RRT is failing the growing number of patients with CKD in developing countries with respect to the benefits presented by KT in helping them return to a near-normal and productive lives [37].

This chapter explores the manifold challenges, innovations, and recommendations for improving KT services in developing countries. Healthcare infrastructure constraints, financial challenged, donor shortages, regulatory and policy concerns, and lack of skilled manpower are among the major obstacles to the advancement of KT. It will also examine a couple of medical and technological advances that can be appropriated to improve organ transplantation success. It will also propose some policy, funding, and capacity-building measures to KT programmes in developing nations.

3. Epidemiology of kidney disease in developing countries

3.1 Prevalence and incidence of CKD and ESRD in developing countries

Although the prevalence of CKD in developing countries is often underreported due to a lack of comprehensive data collection systems, the true incidence rates are estimated to be quadruple that of those seen in developed countries [39, 40]. Factors contributing to this high prevalence include late diagnosis, inadequate healthcare infrastructure, and high rates of risk factors.

Developed nations, with more established healthcare systems, report CKD prevalence rates between 11 and 13%. In contrast, developing countries may experience prevalence rates as high as 20%, with many cases going undiagnosed until the disease has advanced significantly [41]. A World Bank reported that of all the disease groups, CKD accounts for the largest number of people (188 million annually in low-income and lower-middle-income countries) suffering dire health care expenditures worldwide [42].

The incidence of ESRD is on the rise in developing countries. The higher rates of CKD progression, delayed diagnosis, and limited access to early-stage treatment drive this increase.

3.2 Risk factors for CKD and ESRD in developing countries

Hypertension, diabetes mellitus, glomerulonephritis, interstitial nephritis, and congenital abnormalities are the main aetiological for CKD [43]. Blood-borne infections such as chronic hepatitis B and C, and HIV, which are importable causes of CKD, are notoriously prevalent in many developing regions. Exposure to potential nephrotoxins, in heavy metals and agrochemicals, is also more common in developing countries on account of weaker regulatory controls and occupational hazards. The use of traditional herbal medications, which may contain nephrotoxins, is particularly prevalent in many developing countries as a result of cultural practices and limited access to orthodox medicine [4, 44]. Lack of local regulatory oversight and quality control of these products poses a significant risk to health. Importantly, ESRD of unknown cause have been on the rise through the last decades, especially in developing countries [45].

Compounding the various risk factors for CKD and ESRD is poverty. Poverty limits access to health care, healthy food, and clean water, all of which are essential for preventing and managing CKD. Moreover, a lack of education and awareness about kidney disease and its risk factors contributes to late diagnosis and poor management. Public health campaigns and educational programmes are often underfunded and insufficiently widespread.

The epidemiology of kidney disease in developing countries is thus characterized by high and increasing prevalence and incidence rates, driven by common risk factors such as hypertension, diabetes, infections, and environmental exposures.

4. Current status of kidney transplantation in developing countries

Kidney transplantation is widely regarded as the optimal treatment for end-stage renal disease (ESRD), offering improved survival rates and quality of life compared to dialysis. However, various challenges hamper the establishment and success of KT programmes in developing countries. Notwithstanding, there have been significant progress in some regions, indicating the potential for progress with appropriate strategies and interventions.

The availability of specialized transplant units and medical equipment is limited in many developing countries. Urban areas often concentrate these facilities, depriving rural populations of essential transplantation services. The disparity in healthcare infrastructure is a significant barrier to the widespread adoption of kidney transplantation [46].

The availability of national strategies to address CKD has been found to correlate with a country's income level. According to the 2023 Global Kidney Health Atlas [47], only 13% of low-income countries (LIC) have such strategies in place. This percentage increases to 23% in lower-middle-income countries (LMIC) and remains similar at 22% for upper-middle-income countries. In contrast, 33% of high-income countries (HIC) have developed comprehensive national strategies to combat CKD. This data highlights the disparity in CKD management efforts based on economic status, emphasizing the need for targeted support and resources in lower-income regions [47]. In LICs and LMICs, individuals and their family bear most of the health care costs. Only 13% of LICs and 19% of LMICs cover the cost of RRT for adults [48].

The availability of KT services in developing countries varies significantly due to differences in healthcare infrastructure, financial resources, cultural attitudes, and government policies. While some countries have made significant advancements, others are still in the nascent stages of developing their transplantation programs.

In Sub-Saharan Africa, there is a scarcity of KT services. Many patients with end-stage renal disease (ESRD) rely on dialysis due to the lack of transplant centers. Majority of the ESRD patients who can afford KT travel mostly to India, Turkey, and Europe for their operations. When they return to their home countries, management of late surgical complications, and long-term follow-ups may be suboptimal if adequate and timely local medical expertize is not available. That can compromise graft survival and patient outcome. A trend is developing where foreign surgeons and their teams travel to the sub-Saharan African nations to conduct the operations. These "itinerant surgeons" or "surgical merchants" often charge per patient-pair operated on, and skill transfer to the local team may not be a priority. On a brighter note, emerging programmes are starting to change this landscape. For example, Tanzania began offering kidney transplantation services locally in 2017 at Muhimbili National Hospital and Benjamin Mkapa Hospital with international support [5].

In South Asia, India has made significant strides with numerous transplant centers springing across the country. However, access remains uneven, with better services relatively concentrated in urban areas. In contrast, Pakistan and Bangladesh have fewer transplant centers and financial challenges and of trained professionals [6, 7].

In Latin America, Brazil has successfully integrated KT into its public health system and is able to provide transplants free of charge through the Unified Health System. This has resulted in a relatively high number of transplants compared to other developing countries. Similarly, Argentina has a relatively high KT rate but still faces challenges in ensuring equitable access [4, 8].

Egypt has a well-developed KT programme with several specialized centers. However, the prevalence of hepatitis C has historically been a barrier to transplantation [9]. In other countries within the Middle East and North Africa (MENA) region, KT services are rather limited. These countries often rely on international collaboration for training and support. Significant differences exist in the region's capacity to provide RRT, affecting the availability and quality of care [10].

The outcomes of KT in developing countries vary widely due to differences in healthcare infrastructure, availability of resources, and socioeconomic factors. Short-term patient survival rates (one-year post-transplant) in some developing countries, such as India and Brazil, range from 85 to 95%, which are similar to those in high-income countries [11]. However, long-term survival rates (5- and 10-year) are largely lower in developing regions. This difference is mainly due to inadequate access to immunosuppressive drugs, inadequate follow-up care, and higher rates of complications like infections. For example, in Nigeria, five-year graft survival rates are reported to be around 60%, compared to over 70% in developed countries [1, 12].

The status of KT in developing countries is, therefore, marked by significant disparities in infrastructure, expertize, and outcomes compared to developed nations. Despite laudable efforts and achievements in some regions, challenges such as inadequate facilities, financial constraints, and governmental support and commitment exist.

5. Challenges in kidney transplantation in developing countries

In developing countries, KT as a treatment for ESRD faces numerous challenges. These challenges include inadequate medical infrastructure, significant financial constraints, scarcity of donor organs, insufficient regulatory frameworks, and a lack of trained healthcare professionals. Addressing these barriers is essential for improving transplant outcomes and expanding access to this life-saving procedure in resource-limited settings.

5.1 Financial constraints

Healthcare systems in developing countries receive less financial support compared to developed countries, with funding ranging from 0.8–4% of gross national income, while developed countries allocate 10–15% of their gross national income to health care [13, 14, 34].

In general, the low healthcare expenditure is indicative of the availability of various options for RRT. Kidney transplantation appears to be particularly vulnerable to financial challenges, as these challenges affect every stage of the transplantation process. The expenses on KT are incurred at every stage, starting from patient preparation and continuing through the follow-up stage [15–18]. Acquisition and accessibility of consumables and immunosuppression medications are also affected.

5.2 Lack of facilities, equipment, and consumables

The pervasive financial limitations in developing nations hinder the establishment and maintenance of KT programmes. These issues arise from the inability to provide specialized facilities and equipment like dialysis machines and advanced imaging technologies. Immunological and pathological laboratory services are often not up to par [15]. Supply chains for necessary equipment parts, consumables, and immunosuppressive medications are often unreliable. Due to limited local resources, many developing countries rely on external funding and support, which are often inconsistent and unreliable [15].

5.3 Cost of manpower training and retention

Many developing nations, particularly those in the sub-Saharan Africa region, have shortages of nephrologists who possess specialized knowledge in KT [19]. Adequate specialized training in KT (particularly in the surgical operations and nephrology) is mandatory for success of every transplant programme. These professional training are often held in dedicated training programs and at courses and workshops.

Centers with adequate resources (including simulation models), sufficient case volumes, and experience in KT and skill transfer are mostly located in developed countries [20–22]. The financial cost of accessing these training, in terms of travel, lodging, and training fees, can be prohibitive for some countries [23]. Additionally, skilled staff to run the KT services often migrate to developed countries in search of "greener pastures".

5.4 Cost of transplantation and post-operative care

Poor economic status invariably impacts the ability of patients to afford KT. Kidney transplantation is expensive, covering pre-operation evaluation, surgery, immunosuppressive drugs (lifelong), hospitalization, and follow-up care (including management of any complications). Full coverage of all KT costs is available in only 31% of countries globally [15, 24]. Most patients bear these costs out-of-pocket, and the financial burden can lead to impoverishment and hardship for the patient's family. Patients may be compelled to default follow-up and medication appointments following kidney transplantation as a result of these challenges [16].

In developing countries, some centers may choose not to use any induction immunosuppression regimen on account of cost or unavailability [15, 25–27]. The high cost of immunosuppression drugs may prevent patients from maintaining it. This can lead to medication nonadherence and eventual graft loss [28, 29].

Health insurance, where available, often does not cover the full cost of transplantation and associated care, and low penetration of health insurance in many developing countries worsen the problem. Most people find private insurance unaffordable, and public insurance schemes often lack sufficient funds. Government funding for transplant programmes is often inadequate, and dependence on NGOs is unsustainable [30–32].

5.5 Barriers to organ donation

Several factors contribute to the low rates of kidney donation in developing countries, including cultural and religious beliefs, lack of awareness and education, legal and regulatory barriers, and financial concerns.

5.5.1 Cultural and religious beliefs

In many cultures, organ donation is associated with various taboos and superstitions. Some believe that organ donation disrupts the body's integrity and affects the afterlife, considerably hindering donation rates [33]. While some cultures may be more open to living donation within families, they remain hesitant about deceased donation [49]. The decision-making process regarding organ donation is often a collective effort involving families rather than an individual decision. This collective approach may be influenced by cultural practices, societal norms, and family dynamics [50]. Moreover, ethical and professional practices often prioritize these family input and consent.

Religious opposition can also pose a significant barrier. Certain religious beliefs oppose organ donation due to interpretations of religious texts or concerns about the sanctity of the human body [51].For instance, some death rituals or religious ceremonies may conflict with the organ donation process [49].

Cultural and religious beliefs can affect levels of knowledge about organ donation [52]. Misconceptions and fears about organ donation also play a significant role. Common fears include the belief that organ removal violates the sanctity of the deceased, concerns about being cut up after death, the desire to be buried whole, and misconceptions about brain death [53].

5.5.2 Lack of awareness and education

Public awareness about the benefits of organ donation and the process involved is often lacking in developing countries [54]. Many people are unaware that they can donate their organs or do not understand the basic concepts of organ donation. This lack of awareness is compounded by misinformation and myths about organ donation, such as fears of organ trafficking or concerns about the body being mutilated [55]. These misconceptions contribute considerably to the reluctance to donate.

5.5.3 Legal and regulatory barriers

In many regions, the absence of comprehensive legal frameworks governing organ donation and transplantation creates reservations and hinders the establishment of effective donation systems. Regulations that are in place may be poorly enforced, leading to mistrust and reluctance among potential donors and their families [56].

Furthermore, bureaucratic hurdles and protracted approval processes can delay or prevent organ donation and transplantation procedures. This inefficiency not only impacts the timely availability of organs but also discourages individuals from participating in the donation process. Strengthening legal and regulatory structures, ensuring transparency, and streamlining administrative processes are essential steps to overcome these barriers.

5.5.4 Financials concerns

The cost of medical procedures related to organ donation, including hospital stays, surgical procedures, and post-operative care, can be too high for many families. Even when donation is altruistic, the associated expenses can discourage potential donors. Moreover, the lack of financial incentives or compensation for living donors adds to the challenge. In many cases, donors may face loss of income due to time taken off work for the donation process and recovery period. Instituting policies that provide some financial support and incentives for donors, as well as covering medical expenses, could appreciably boost donation rates [57].

5.6 Regulatory and policy issues

Many developing countries lack national KT programmes and registries, which are essential for directing and monitoring transplantation activities. Inefficient regulatory structures can create barriers to the smooth operation of KT programmes, including cumbersome bureaucratic processes and a lack of clear guidelines for transplantation practices [15].

Legal and ethical issues further complicate the landscape of KT in developing countries. The prevalence of commercial organ trade undermines ethical standards and can lead to the exploitation of vulnerable populations. This practice is often a result of weak regulatory frameworks and lack of enforcement [15, 58]. Additionally, high medicolegal responsibilities and potential psychosocial burdens associated with

KT practice can deter medical professionals from participating in transplantation programmes [31].

Policy and legislative gaps also pose significant challenges. Many developing countries lack the requisite legislation that supports organ donation and transplantation. This includes laws that define brain death, regulate organ procurement, and ensure ethical standards in transplantation practices [59]. In the absence of these legislation, it becomes difficult to establish a structured and reliable system for organ donation and transplantation.

6. Strategies for improvement

6.1 Human capacity development

6.1.1 Establishment of academic programs

Established transplant programmes in academic centers in developing countries should develop structured fellowship programs for physicians, surgeons, and nurses, covering both theoretical knowledge and practical skills. These programmes should include, among others, curriculum covering pre-transplant evaluation, donor selection, surgical techniques, post-transplant care, and immunosuppression management. The programmes should also provide for hands-on clinical experience with a minimum number of transplant cases. When these centers align with regional specialty colleges, training of specialists from other centers and neighboring countries can be facilitated. It would be prudent for research to be a core mandate of such programmes.

6.1.2 International partnership and mentoring

Collaboration with established transplant centers and organizations in other countries is vital for providing training opportunities, mentorship, and knowledge transfer. The Transplant Links Community (TLC) has successfully implemented this approach. TLC provides hands-on surgical mentoring, lectures, and training seminars at partner units in developing countries, along with continuous long-term support [19]. Transplant centers in teaching hospitals can seek mentorship and training support from these organizations in developed countries. Engaging these mentor institutions is more economically viable, as their assistance is often not financially motivated. Furthermore, because these institutions possess the full range of skills and knowledge required for KT, they can provide comprehensive multidisciplinary training for the entire local team. This approach contrasts with engaging a single transplant surgeon proctor without the support of other specialists, such as nephrologists. Inadequate training for the nephrology team can negatively impact patient outcomes.

6.1.3 International fellowship and observership training

Surgical skill acquisition through proctorship can be prolonged because operations with proctors are often scheduled infrequently, requiring alignment of the local team's schedule with that of the proctor. It takes longer for local surgeons to gain the confidence needed to operate independently. Even skilled surgeons who perform more complex surgeries than kidney transplantation must navigate the small margin of error inherent in these procedures. Complications arising from surgical mishaps can be disastrous and demoralize the local team, eroding confidence among potential recipients and donors.

Thus, it is imperative for local surgeons to have extensive exposure to kidney transplant operations. This exposure will boost their confidence and that of the team and potential patients. Ideally, training should occur in high-volume kidney transplant centers, providing hands-on experience. If hands-on training is not available, observing a variety of cases, managing intraoperative and postoperative complications, and learning from these experiences can offer valuable lessons that would otherwise take more time and potentially lead to adverse patient outcomes.

6.1.4 *Training and continuous medical education programmes*

Training programmes for nephrologists, transplant surgeons, nurses, and other healthcare professionals involved in KT should be created. These programmes should foster collaboration among the various sub-specialties and be tailored to the specific challenges and available resources locally. Some of these programs can be accessed from charity organizations such as the TLC [60].

Ongoing continuous medical education (CME) programmes to keep healthcare professionals updated on the latest advancements and best practices in KT should be organized, leveraging online platforms and telemedicine to expand access to training resources and expert consultations. Training programmes should also carry out regular evaluations and competency assessments to ensure training programs meet international standards.

6.2 Public-private partnerships

Public-private partnerships (PPPs) can play an important role in advancing KT in developing countries. These partnerships can help address resource constraints, improve infrastructure, and enhance the quality of care.

PPPs can be appropriated for the establishment of dialysis centers that can create a foundation for expanding into transplantation services [61]. PPPs can help build or refurbish healthcare facilities dedicated to KT ensuring sustainability and high standards. This model has been successful in various healthcare sectors and can be applied to transplant centers [62]. Partnerships can also bring in private sector expertize to improve clinical services related to KT. This can include training programmes, quality improvement initiatives, and introduction of new technologies. Facility management, IT support, and logistics can be outsourced to private sector partners, allowing healthcare professionals to focus on clinical care.

PPPs can facilitate steady supply of immunosuppressive drugs at subsidized and affordable prices for transplant success [63]. Innovative financing models through PPPs can also help make kidney transplantation more accessible and affordable in resource-poor settings [1].

6.3 Policy advocacy

Policy advocacy and changes can help accelerate KT in developing countries.

Developing effective national strategies for CKD is essential in that regard. These strategies should cover prevention, early diagnosis, and treatment of kidney disease, along with provisions for KT. Countries need to create CKD-specific policies that directly address organ procurement, allocation, and post-transplant care. This will ensure fair and transparent organ allocation systems to comply with acceptable ethical transplantation practices [1, 64].

To tackle organ trafficking and protect vulnerable populations, policies must be applied to curtail transplant tourism and prevent commercialization. Countries should also consider adopting opt-in or opt-out organ donation policies that best align with their cultural contexts and healthcare systems. Comprehensive legal frameworks are necessary to support organ donation and transplantation, including clear guidelines on donor consent, organ allocation, and ethical practices. Establishing national donor registries as well as independent regulatory bodies can streamline the organ matching process, ensure transparency, and prevent illegal activities [6, 65].

Incorporating KT into universal health coverage schemes will improve access and affordability. Policies should aim to, as much as possible, reduce out-of-pocket expenses for transplant recipients and living donors, providing financial and non-financial incentives to encourage organ donation. This includes covering medical expenses, offering recognition programs, and implementing compensation schemes for living donors to cover lost wages and travel costs. Comprehensive post-donation care and follow-up, including medical, psychological, and social support, should also be ensured [66].

6.4 Community education and engagement

Community engagement is an essential strategy for improving KT outcomes in developing countries. It provides a unique avenue to address cultural, social, and logistical barriers to transplantation. Collaborative community-engaged approaches also help to identify and address specific barriers to KT. This involves working with key stakeholders, patients, and healthcare providers to develop tailored interventions [67].

Raising awareness about kidney disease and transplantation through community education programmes and public education campaigns can help dispel myths, reduce stigma, and increase the willingness to donate organs. These campaigns should be culturally sensitive and use local languages, employing various media platforms, including radio, television, social media, and print media, to reach diverse audiences [68]. Engaging celebrities and influencers to endorse organ donation can leverage their reach and impact, while tailoring messages to align with cultural and religious values ensures respectful and effective communication. Sharing testimonials from donors and recipients can humanize the subject, build empathy, and support, and highlighting success stories and positive outcomes of organ transplantation can inspire and motivate potential donors. At a higher level, organ donation education can be integrated into school curricula and community programs to foster a culture of donation from an early age. Facilitating interfaith dialogs can address religious concerns and misconceptions about organ donation [69].

Including patients and their families in the decision-making process ensures that their perspectives and preferences are considered, improving adherence to treatment plans and increasing satisfaction with care [68]. Training and employing community health workers (CHWs) can bridge the gap between healthcare providers and the community. CHWs can provide education, support, and follow-up care, especially in rural or underserved areas [69].

These strategies will enable healthcare providers to engage communities more effectively, address barriers to kidney transplantation, and eventually improve outcomes for patients in developing countries.

6.5 Technological and medical innovations

6.5.1 Telemedicine and e-health

Telemedicine and e-health technologies offer major potential to enhance KT programmes in developing countries. These innovations can help circumvent geographical, financial, and logistical barriers, thereby improving access to care and patient outcomes. They also facilitate capacity building and training, making them essential tools in modern healthcare delivery.

One of the primary strategies for leveraging telemedicine and e-health in kidney transplantation is through remote monitoring and follow-up care. Telemedicine facilitates continuous monitoring of KT patients, reducing the need for frequent in-person visits. This is particularly beneficial for patients residing in remote areas with limited access to transplant centers. The application of telemedicine for remote monitoring has proven numerous benefits, including reduced travel time and costs, better adherence to medications, and more reliable blood pressure control [70].

Video conferencing tools further enhance this by enabling real-time consultations between patients and transplant specialists. Additionally, asynchronous communication platforms allow patients to upload their medical records and symptoms for later review by specialists. These teleconsultations have been successfully used to provide chronic care for transplant recipients, demonstrating both safety and high patient satisfaction [71].

Educational resources and self-management tools can also be deployed through e-health platforms. These platforms empower patients by providing access to medication reminders, symptom tracking, and educational materials about post-transplant care. Studies have shown that e-health solutions improve the quality of life, physical function, and overall health among transplant patients. By enabling patients to participate actively in their care, these platforms contribute to better health outcomes and increased patient engagement [72].

Capacity building and training can also be enhanced through telemedicine and e-health. These technologies facilitate the training of healthcare professionals and enable the conduct of multidisciplinary team meetings. This ensures that all team members are up to date with the latest protocols and practices, ultimately leading to better patient outcomes. Telemedicine and e-health also provide opportunities for continuous professional development, essential for maintaining high standards of care in kidney transplantation.

6.5.2 Medical advances

Innovative medical advancements have the potential to improve KT outcomes in developing countries. These advancements include minimally invasive techniques, enhanced immunosuppressive therapies, and advanced organ preservation methods.

6.5.2.1 Minimally invasive techniques

Minimally invasive techniques, such as laparoscopic donor nephrectomy, have shown considerable benefits in kidney transplantation. This technique reduces hospital stays and recovery time, minimizes surgical trauma and post-op pain, and decreases overall costs. Training surgeons in laparoscopic techniques can be cost-effective and improve patient outcomes. Centers of excellence where these techniques can be practiced and perfected should be created. This should go in tandem with investment in cost-effective laparoscopic equipment, instruments, and consumables suitable for resource-limited settings.

6.5.2.2 Advancements in immunosuppressive therapy

The availability of generic immunosuppressive drugs, such as tacrolimus and mycophenolate mofetil, has reduced costs while maintaining efficacy. Studies have shown that generic formulations of immunosuppressive drugs are effective and safe for transplant patients. For instance, research by Belin et al. has demonstrated that generic immunosuppressive regimens are effective for KT maintenance therapy, providing a cost-effective alternative to branded drugs while maintaining clinical efficacy [73]. Governments and hospitals can negotiate bulk purchases to further lower costs.

6.5.2.3 Hypothermic machine perfusion (HMP)

Hypothermic machine perfusion has been shown to significantly improve the viability of kidney allografts, especially from marginal donors, by reducing complications and increasing graft survival. Studies have shown that HMP helps in maintaining cellular integrity and reducing ischemia-reperfusion injury, which is critical for the success KT. Though the initial cost of the HMP setup may be costly, its use can be cost-effective in the long run due to better outcomes and reduced need for retransplantation. The reduced incidence of complications and improved long-term graft function translate into lower overall healthcare costs, making HMP a financially viable option for kidney preservation [74].

6.6 Development and adoption of cost-effective technologies and medical devices

6.6.1 Low-cost dialysis machines

One of the important needs in KT is the availability of affordable dialysis machines. Developing and distributing portable dialysis units that are easy to use in remote and resource-limited settings can be lifesaving for patients awaiting transplantation. Encouraging local manufacturing of dialysis machines can further reduce costs and ensure a steady supply.

6.6.2 Affordable diagnostic tools

Point-of-care (POC) diagnostic tools are essential for rapid and accurate monitoring of important parameters such as blood creatinine levels, electrolyte balance, and drug concentrations. These tools are especially vital in resource-limited settings where access to advanced laboratory facilities may be limited. POC diagnostics can significantly improve early detection of complications and timely interventions, thereby improving patient outcomes [75, 76].

6.6.3 Sustainable medical devices

The promotion of high-quality reusable medical instruments can help lower costs and reliance on single-use items. Proper sterilization protocols must, however, be established to maintain safety standards. Investment in reliable autoclaves and sterilization units is essential to ensure the safe reuse of the medical instruments. Additionally, training healthcare staff on the maintenance and safe use of reusable instruments is important for sustaining these practices.

6.6.4 Mobile health applications

Mobile health (mHealth) applications offer numerous potential benefits for transplant patients by providing medication reminders, educational resources, and communication channels with healthcare providers. These apps can enhance patient engagement, adherence to treatment plans, and self-management, particularly in remote areas with limited access to healthcare facilities. The integration of mHealth applications into patient care can lead to improved health outcomes and better management of chronic conditions [77, 78].

Adopting and integrating technological and medical innovations can prove crucial for advancing KT in developing countries. Telemedicine and e-health can bridge gaps in specialist care and continuous monitoring, while recent medical advances in minimally invasive techniques and immunosuppression can improve patient outcomes. Additionally, the development and adoption of affordable technologies and medical devices can make KT more accessible and sustainable in resource-limited settings.

7. Case studies and success stories

7.1 Case Study: Sindh Institute of Urology and Transplantation (SIUT)

The Sindh Institute of Urology and Transplantation (SIUT) in Pakistan provides an excellent model of how developing countries can establish successful kidney transplantation programs. In the 1980s, SIUT developed a combined dialysis and living-related KT programme within the government sector. The institute operates on a distinctive community–government partnership, where funding is shared between the community and the government (40–60%). All services, including dialysis, transplantation, and lifelong follow-up care with medications, are provided free of cost to patients. This approach ensures comprehensive care for ESRD patients, addressing the shortage of deceased donor organs by focusing on living-related transplants.

The SIUT model has proven self-sustaining for over 25 years. The institute serves over 600 dialysis patients daily and performs 7 to10 living-related transplants weekly. As of 2018, SIUT had conducted 9150 transplants, achieving 1-year and 5-year graft survival rates of 92% and 85%, respectively. SIUT's success has established it as a center of excellence for renal transplantation in Pakistan and has significantly influenced national policies against transplant tourism and in support of transplant laws.

By leveraging community–government partnerships, providing integrated and cost-effective care, and influencing national transplantation policies, SIUT has significantly improved access to kidney transplantation for a large segment of the marginalized population in Pakistan.

7.2 Case study: Fortis Hospital in India

Fortis Hospital is a leading healthcare provider in India, renowned for its advanced KT programme. The hospital has achieved major success in providing high-quality care and excellent outcomes for kidney transplant patients. Central to this success is a comprehensive approach that encompasses pre-transplant evaluations, innovative surgical techniques, and robust post-transplant care.

At Fortis Hospital, the pre-transplant evaluation process is thorough and meticulous. It includes blood tests for human leukocyte antigen (HLA) matching, viral serology, biochemistry analysis, and radiology evaluations. The multidisciplinary team at Fortis Hospital is a core component of its successful transplantation programme, ensuring that patients receive holistic care tailored to their specific needs.

Fortis Hospital also uses advanced technologies and surgical techniques to improve the success rates of kidney transplants. Post-operative care at Fortis Hospital involves continuous monitoring and support for patients, with a focus on immunosuppressive medication management and prompt care of any complications that may arise. The success of Fortis Hospital's kidney transplantation program has been attributed to its highly skilled team, advanced infrastructure, and patient-centered care. By focusing on individualized care and providing comprehensive support for patients and their families, Fortis Hospital has set a benchmark for kidney transplantation programs in developing countries. Their model shows that with structured and comprehensive approaches, high-quality care and excellent outcomes are achievable, offering valuable lessons for other healthcare systems aiming to improve their transplantation services.

7.3 Case study: Hospital do Rim in Brazil

Hospital do Rim (HRim) in São Paulo, Brazil, stands out as a world leader in kidney transplantation. Over an 18-year period, the hospital had performed more than 11,496 kidney transplants, making it one of the highest-volume transplant centers globally. The hospital's success can be attributed to its innovative "assembly line" approach to kidney transplantation, which has streamlined processes, increased efficiency, and standardized care. This high-volume transplant program allows the hospital to perform over 1000 transplants annually, ensuring timely and effective treatment for many patients. The clinical outcomes at Hospital do Rim are exemplary, with five-year graft survival rates of 91.1% for living donors and 79.7% for deceased donors.

Several factors contribute to the success of Hospital do Rim. The hospital's structured approach to transplantation has optimized resource utilization and significantly improved patient outcomes. Their relentless focus on high-quality care and maintaining rigorous standards as well as ongoing research initiatives have been pivotal to the program's achievements [79, 80].

7.4 Case study: Groote Schuur Hospital in South Africa

Groote Schuur Hospital in Cape Town, South Africa, is a renowned public academic hospital known for its innovative KT programme, serving a diverse population. A major component of the hospital's programme is its robust deceased donor program, which adopts a liberal approach to donor selection by utilizing extended criteria donors (ECD) and donors after circulatory death (DCD). This strategy has significantly expanded the donor pool.

Groote Schuur hospital has also pioneered HIV positive-to-positive kidney transplants and expanded the donor pool further and provided life-saving treatments to

HIV-positive patients. The hospital's comprehensive care model ensures continuous and integrated care, including acute and chronic dialysis services, pre-transplant evaluations, and post-transplant follow-ups.

Groote Schuur Hospital exemplifies how a public academic institution can achieve excellence in kidney transplantation through innovation, equity, and comprehensive care. By leveraging strong institutional support and adopting innovative practices, Groote Schuur has significantly improved KT outcomes and set a benchmark for other institutions in resource-limited settings [44, 81].

The case studies of Sindh Institute of Urology and Transplantation (SIUT) in Pakistan, Fortis Hospital in India, Hospital do Rim in Brazil, and Groote Schuur Hospital in South Africa demonstrate that successful kidney transplantation programs can be established in developing countries through innovative approaches, comprehensive care models, and strong institutional support.

8. Conclusion

This chapter has examined the critical challenges and innovative strategies essential for advancing kidney transplantation in developing countries. The journey toward improving transplantation outcomes in these regions is fraught with significant obstacles, yet ripe with opportunities for impactful solutions.

One of the primary challenges lies in the inadequate medical and healthcare infrastructure. Many developing countries lack the specialized facilities and equipment necessary for high-quality kidney transplantation, which directly affects the accessibility and effectiveness of these services. Financial constraints further complicate this issue, as the high costs associated with transplantation and post-operative care, coupled with limited funding and insurance coverage, create formidable barriers for patients and healthcare providers alike.

The lack of donor organs is another major hurdle. Cultural and religious beliefs, along with a general lack of awareness and inadequate legal frameworks, significantly contribute to the low rates of organ donation. This scarcity is compounded by insufficient training and capacity-building opportunities for healthcare professionals, which undermines the effectiveness of transplantation programs. Additionally, inefficient organizational oversight and gaps in policy and legislation add layers of complexity to the establishment and maintenance of successful kidney transplantation initiatives.

Addressing these challenges requires a multifaceted approach. Building capacity through training programs and centers of excellence is vital for enhancing the skills and knowledge of healthcare professionals. Public-private partnerships can play a crucial role in improving access to transplantation services and sharing resources efficiently. Policy advocacy is essential to promote legal frameworks that facilitate organ donation and address regulatory barriers, while community engagement efforts can significantly boost public awareness and donor rates by addressing cultural and educational gaps.

Innovative solutions are equally important in overcoming these challenges. The use of telemedicine and e-health for remote monitoring and follow-up care can reduce costs and enhance access to specialist care. Minimally invasive techniques, such as laparoscopic procedures, can improve patient outcomes by reducing recovery times. Advancements in immunosuppressive therapy, including the use of generic drugs, can make post-transplant care more affordable. Hypothermic machine perfusion offers promising improvements in organ preservation and graft survival rates. Additionally, developing affordable technologies, such as low-cost dialysis machines and diagnostic tools, can make kidney care more accessible in resource-limited settings.

In summary, by addressing the multi-layered challenges with strategic and innovative solutions, developing countries can significantly enhance their kidney transplantation programs. These efforts will lead to better patient outcomes, increased access to life-saving treatments, and a more sustainable and effective healthcare system for kidney disease management.

9. Future directions

To further advance KT in developing countries, a strategic focus on research, policy, and practical implementation is essential. Future efforts should prioritize research into innovative techniques and technologies, such as minimally invasive surgical methods and advanced immunosuppressive therapies, to improve patient outcomes and reduce costs. Additionally, region-specific studies on the epidemiology of kidney disease can help tailor programs to local needs, while robust data collection systems can track transplant outcomes and identify areas for improvement.

Policy initiatives must include the development of comprehensive legal frameworks that support organ donation and transplantation, clearly defining brain death and ethical standards. Sustainable funding models, incorporating public–private partnerships, are crucial for the financial viability of transplant programs. National public awareness campaigns can educate the public about the benefits of organ donation and address cultural and religious concerns, thereby increasing donor rates.

On a practical level, investing in the training and development of healthcare professionals is vital to ensure they possess the necessary skills and knowledge for effective transplantation practices. Leveraging telemedicine and e-health solutions can provide remote monitoring and support for transplant patients, especially in rural areas. Furthermore, engaging local communities in the planning and implementation of transplant programs ensures cultural sensitivity and enhances acceptance.

By focusing on these strategic areas, developing countries can create a more favorable environment for kidney transplantation, leading to better patient outcomes and expanded access to life-saving treatments.

DOI: http://dx.doi.org/10.5772/intechopen.1006699

Author details

Ernest Kwame Adjepong-Tandoh
Korle Bu Teaching Hospital, Accra, Ghana

*Address all correspondence to: adjepongtandoh@yahoo.com

References

[1] Jha V, Garcia-Garcia G, Iseki K, Li Z, Naicker S, Plattner B, et al. Chronic kidney disease: Global dimension and perspectives. Lancet [Internet]. 2013;**382**(9888):260-272. Available from: https://pubmed.ncbi.nlm.nih.gov/23727169/

[2] George C, Mogueo A, Okpechi I, Echouffo-Tcheugui JB, Kengne AP. Chronic kidney disease in low-income to middle-income countries: The case for increased screening. BMJ Global Health [Internet]. 2017;**2**(2):e000256. Available from: https://gh.bmj.com/content/2/2/e000256

[3] Jager KJ, Kovesdy C, Langham R, Rosenberg M, Jha V, Zoccali C. A single number for advocacy and communication-worldwide more than 850 million individuals have kidney diseases. Kidney International [Internet]. 2019;**96**(5):1048-1050. Available from: http://www.ncbi.nlm.nih.gov/pubmed/31582227

[4] Ulasi II, Awobusuyi O, Nayak S, Ramachandran R, Musso CG, Depine SA, et al. Chronic kidney disease burden in low-resource settings: Regional perspectives. Seminars in Nephrology [Internet]. 2022;**42**(5):1-12. Available from: https://pubmed.ncbi.nlm.nih.gov/37058859/

[5] Furia FF, Shoo J, Ruggajo PJ, Kilonzo K, Basu G, Yeates K, et al. Developing nephrology services in low income countries: A case of Tanzania. BMC Nephrology [Internet]. 2019;**20**(1):1-8. Available from: https://pubmed.ncbi.nlm.nih.gov/31623570/

[6] Garcia GG, Harden P, Chapman J. The global role of kidney transplantation. Kidney & Blood Pressure Research [Internet]. 2012;**35**(5):299-304. DOI: 10.1159/000337044

[7] Ullah K, Dogar AW, Ochani S, Shoaib A, Shah HH, Ur Rehman ME. Obstacles to the Deceased Donor Transplantation in Pakistan. Vol. 10. BMJ Open Gastroenterology: BMJ Publishing Group; 2023

[8] More than 12,000 organ transplants were performed in Brazil between January and November in 2021 [Internet]. Available from: https://www.gov.br/en/government-of-brazil/latest-news/2022/more-than-12-000-organ-transplants-were-performed-in-brazil-between-january-and-november-in-2021 [Accessed: July 23, 2024]

[9] Egypt establishes largest center for organ transplantation in Middle East: Minister - Egypt Independent [Internet]. Available from: https://www.egyptindependent.com/egypt-establishes-largest-center-for-organ-transplantation-in-middle-east-minister/ [Accessed: July 23, 2024]

[10] Rashidi MM, Moghaddam SS, Azadnajafabad S, Mohammadi E, Khalaji A, Malekpour MR, et al. Mortality and disability-adjusted life years in North Africa and Middle East attributed to kidney dysfunction: A systematic analysis for the global burden of disease study 2019. Clinical Kidney Journal [Internet]. 2023;**17**(1):1-13. Available from: https://pubmed.ncbi.nlm.nih.gov/38288035/

[11] Garcia GC, Harden P, Chapman J. The global role of kidney transplantation. Transplantation. 2012;**93**:337-341

[12] Arogundade FA. Kidney transplantation in a low-resource setting: Nigeria experience. Kidney International Supplements (2011) [Internet].

2013;**3**(2):241. Available from: /pmc/articles/PMC4089648/ [Accessed: July 23, 2024]

[13] Siraj MS. Deceased organ transplantation in Bangladesh: The dynamics of bioethics, religion and culture. HEC Forum [Internet]. 2022;**34**(2):139-167. Available from: https://pubmed.ncbi.nlm.nih.gov/33595774/

[14] Rizvi SAH, Naqvi SAA, Zafar MN, Hussain Z, Hashmi A, Hussain M, et al. A renal transplantation model for developing countries. American Journal of Transplantation. 2011;**11**(11):2302-2307

[15] Gadelkareem RA, Abdelgawad AM, Mohammed N, Zarzour MA, Khalil M, Reda A, et al. Challenges to establishing and maintaining kidney transplantation programs in developing countries: What are the coping strategies? World Journal of Methodology [Internet]. 2024;**14**(2):1-11. Available from: /pmc/articles/PMC11229866/

[16] Venkataraman S, Kendrick J. Barriers to kidney transplantation in ESKD. Seminars in Dialysis [Internet]. 2020;**33**(6):523-532. Available from: https://pubmed.ncbi.nlm.nih.gov/33015941/

[17] Kasiske BL, London W, Ellison MD. Race and socioeconomic factors influencing early placement on the kidney transplant waiting list. Journal of the American Society of Nephrology: JASN. 1998;**9**(11):2142-2147. Available from: https://pubmed.ncbi.nlm.nih.gov/9808103/

[18] Goldfarb-Rumyantzev AS, Koford JK, Baird BC, Chelamcharla M, Habib AN, Wang BJ, et al. Role of socioeconomic status in kidney transplant outcome. Clinical Journal of the American Society of Nephrology [Internet]. 2006;**1**(2):313-322. Available from: https://pubmed.ncbi.nlm.nih.gov/17699222/

[19] Ready AR, Nath J, Milford DV, Adu D, Jewitt-Harris J. Establishing Sustainable Kidney Transplantation Programs in Developing World Countries: A 10-Year Experience. Vol. 90. Kidney International. New York, NY, USA: Elsevier; 2016. pp. 916-920

[20] Cabello R, González C, Quicios C, Bueno G, García JV, Arribas AB, et al. An experimental model for training in renal transplantation surgery with human cadavers preserved using W. Thiel's embalming technique. Journal of Surgical Education [Internet]. 2015;**72**(2):192-197. Available from: https://pubmed.ncbi.nlm.nih.gov/25555672/

[21] Melkonian V, Huy T, Varma CR, Nazzal M, Randall HB, Nguyen MTJ. The creation of a novel low-cost bench-top kidney transplant surgery simulator and a survey on its fidelity and educational utility. Cureus [Internet]. 2020;**12**(11):1-10. Available from: https://pubmed.ncbi.nlm.nih.gov/33312823/

[22] Patnaik R, Khan MTA, Oh T, Yamaguchi S, Fritze DM. Technical skills simulation in transplant surgery: A systematic review. Global Surgical Education - Journal of the Association for Surgical Education [Internet]. 2022;**1**(1):42. Available from: /pmc/articles/PMC9483372/

[23] Hernández D, Caballero A. Kidney transplant in the next decade: Strategies, challenges and vision of the future. Nefrología [Internet]. 2023;**43**(3):281-292. Available from: https://pubmed.ncbi.nlm.nih.gov/37635014/

[24] Mudiayi D, Shojai S, Okpechi I, Christie EA, Wen K, Kamaleldin M, et al. Global estimates of capacity for kidney

transplantation in world countries and regions. Transplantation [Internet]. 2022;**106**(6):1113-1122. Available from: /pmc/articles/PMC9128615/

[25] Babloyan S, Voskanyan M, Shekherdimian S, Nazaryan H, Arakelyan S, Kurkchyan K, et al. Kidney transplantation in low- to middle-income countries: Outcomes and lessons learned from Armenia. Annals of Transplantation [Internet]. 2021;**26**:e930943-1. Available from: /pmc/articles/PMC8464179/

[26] John EE, Mehta S, Sohal PM, Sandhu JS. Predictors of short-term outcomes in living donor renal allograft recipients: A prospective study from a tertiary Care Center in North India. Cureus [Internet]. 2022;**14**(8):1-12. Available from: /pmc/articles/PMC9501959/

[27] Hada R, Prasad N, ABIJ of, 2017 undefined. Outcome of live donor kidney transplantation in a Government Hospital of Nepal. [Internet]. Available from: https://journals.lww.com/ijjt/fulltext/2017/11020/Outcome_of_Live_Donor_Kidney_Transplantation_in_a.7.aspx

[28] Gaynor JJ, Guerra G, Roth D, Chen L, Kupin W, Mattiazzi A, et al. Graft failure due to nonadherence among 150 prospectively-followed kidney transplant recipients at 18 years post-transplant: Our results and review of the literature. Journal of Clinical Medicine [Internet]. 2022;**11**(5):2-16. Available from: http://www.ncbi.nlm.nih.gov/pubmed/35268424

[29] Gordon EJ, Prohaska TR, Gallant MP, Siminoff LA. Adherence to immunosuppression: A prospective diary study. Transplantation Proceedings [Internet]. 2007;**39**(10):3081. Available from: /pmc/articles/PMC2361155/

[30] Amaya-Lara JL. Catastrophic expenditure due to out-of-pocket health payments and its determinants in Colombian households. International Journal for Equity in Health [Internet]. 2016;**15**(1):1-11. Available from: /pmc/articles/PMC5105279/

[31] Essue BM, Laba TL, Knaul F, Chu A, Van, Minh H, Nguyen TKP, et al. Economic burden of chronic ill health and injuries for households in low- and middle-income countries. In: Jamison DT, Gelband H, Horton S, et al., editors. Disease Control Priorities: Improving Health and Reducing Poverty. 3rd ed. Washington, DC: The International Bank for Reconstruction and Development / The World Bank; 27 Nov 2017

[32] Rahman MM, Gilmour S, Saito E, Sultana P, Shibuya K. Health-related financial catastrophe, inequality and chronic illness in Bangladesh. PLoS One [Internet]. 2013;**8**(2):1-7. Available from: /pmc/articles/PMC3581555/

[33] Li MT, Hillyer GC, Husain SA, Mohan S. Cultural barriers to organ donation among Chinese and Korean individuals in the United States: A systematic review. Transplant International [Internet]. 2019;**32**(10):1001. Available from: /pmc/articles/PMC6867085/

[34] Arogundade FA, Omotoso BA, Adelakun A, Bamikefa T, Ezeugonwa R, Omosule B, et al. Burden of end-stage renal disease in sub-Saharan Africa. Clinical Nephrology. 2020;**93**(1):S3-S7

[35] Lalji R, Francis A, Johnson DW, McCulloch M. Health disparities in access to kidney replacement therapy amongst children and adolescents with end-stage kidney disease in low- and lower-middle-income countries. Kidney International [Internet]. 2020;**97**(3):463-465. Available

from: https://pubmed.ncbi.nlm.nih.gov/32008803/

[36] Thurlow JS, Joshi M, Yan G, Norris KC, Agodoa LY, Yuan CM, et al. Global epidemiology of end-stage kidney disease and disparities in kidney replacement therapy. American Journal of Nephrology [Internet]. 2021;**52**(2):98-107. Available from: https://pubmed.ncbi.nlm.nih.gov/33752206/

[37] Ready A, Jewitt-Harris J. Setting-up and running a renal transplant unit. In: Harber M, editor. Primer on Nephrology. 2nd ed. Cham, Switzerland: Springer Nature Switzerland AG; 2022. pp. 1445-1457

[38] Aviles-Gomez R, Luquin-Arellano VH, Garcia-Garcia G, Ibarra-Hernandez M, Briseño-Renteria G. Is renal replacement therapy for all possible in developing countries? Ethnicity & Disease. 2006;**16**(2 Suppl. 2):S2-82-S2-70

[39] Stanifer JW, Jing B, Tolan S, Helmke N, Mukerjee R, Naicker S, et al. The epidemiology of chronic kidney disease in sub-Saharan Africa: A systematic review and meta-analysis. The Lancet Global Health [Internet]. 2014;**2**(3):e174-e181. Available from: https://pubmed.ncbi.nlm.nih.gov/25102850/

[40] Stanifer JW, Muiru A, Jafar TH, Patel UD. Chronic kidney disease in low- and middle-income countries. Nephrology, Dialysis, Transplantation [Internet]. 2016;**31**(6):868-874. Available from: https://pubmed.ncbi.nlm.nih.gov/27217391/

[41] Hill NR, Fatoba ST, Oke JL, Hirst JA, O'Callaghan CA, Lasserson DS, et al. Global prevalence of chronic kidney disease – A systematic review and meta-analysis. PLoS One [Internet]. 2016;**11**(7):e0158765. Available from: https://journals.plos.org/plosone/article?id=10.1371/journal.pone.0158765

[42] Jamison DT, Gelband H, Horton S, Jha P, Laxminarayan R, Mock CN, et al. Disease control priorities: Improving health and reducing poverty. 3rd ed. Washington, DC: The International Bank for Reconstruction and Development / The World Bank; 27 Nov 2017

[43] Barsoum RS. Burden of chronic kidney disease: North Africa. Kidney International Supplements (2011) [Internet]. 2013;**3**(2):164-166. Available from: https://pubmed.ncbi.nlm.nih.gov/25018981/

[44] Davidson B, Du TT, Jones ESW, Barday Z, Manning K, Curdie FM, et al. Outcomes and challenges of a kidney transplant programme at Groote Schuur Hospital, Cape Town: A South African perspective. PLoS One [Internet]. 2019;**14**(1):1-15. Available from: https://pubmed.ncbi.nlm.nih.gov/30682138/

[45] Fiseha T, Osborne NJ. Burden of end-stage renal disease of undetermined etiology in Africa. Renal Replacement Therapy [Internet]. 2023;**9**(1):1-10. Available from: https://rrtjournal.biomedcentral.com/articles/10.1186/s41100-023-00497-w

[46] Naicker S. End-Stage Renal Disease in Sub-Saharan and South Africa. Kidney International, Supplement. 2003;(83):S119-S122. DOI: 10.1046/j.1523-1755.63.s83.25.x

[47] Bello AK, Levin A, Tonelli M, Okpechi IG, Feehally J, Harris D, et al. Assessment of global kidney health care status. JAMA - Journal of the American Medical Association. 2017;**317**(18):1864-1881

[48] Bello AK, Alrukhaimi M, Ashuntantang GE, Bellorin-Font E, Benghanem Gharbi M, Braam B, et al. Global overview of health systems oversight and financing for kidney care. Kidney International Supplements (2011) [Internet]. 2018;**8**(2):41-51. Available from: https://pubmed.ncbi.nlm.nih.gov/30675438/

[49] Doerry K, Oh J, Vincent D, Fischer L, Schulz-Jürgensen S. Religious and cultural aspects of organ donation: Narrowing the gap through understanding different religious beliefs. Pediatric Transplantation [Internet]. 2022;**26**(7):e14339. DOI: 10.1111/petr.14339

[50] Walker W, Broderick A, Sque M. Factors influencing bereaved families' decisions about organ donation: An integrative literature review. Western Journal of Nursing Research. 2013;**35**(10):1339-1359

[51] Oliver M, Woywodt A, Ahmed A, Saif I. Organ donation, transplantation and religion. Nephrology Dialysis Transplantation [Internet]. 2011;**26**(2):437-444. DOI: 10.1093/ndt/gfq628

[52] Oluyombo R, Fawale MB, Ojewola RW, Busari OA, Ogunmola OJ, Olanrewaju TO, et al. Knowledge regarding organ donation and willingness to donate among health workers in South-West Nigeria. International Journal of Organ Transplantation Medicine [Internet]. 2016;**7**(1):19 Available from: /pmc/articles/PMC4756261/

[53] Woo KT. Social and Cultural Aspects of Organ Donation in Asia. BRL:KIE/41147

[54] Mithra P, Ravindra P, Unnikrishnan B, Rekha T, Kanchan T, Kumar N, et al. Perceptions and attitudes towards organ donation among people seeking healthcare in tertiary care centers of coastal South India. Indian Journal of Palliative Care [Internet]. 2013;**19**(2):83. Available from: /pmc/articles/PMC3775029/

[55] Matesanz R, Domínguez-Gil B, Coll E, De La Rosa G, Marazuela R. Spanish experience as a leading country: What kind of measures were taken? Transplant International [Internet]. 2011;**24**(4):333-343. Available from: https://pubmed.ncbi.nlm.nih.gov/21210863/

[56] Budiani-Saberi DA, Delmonico FL. Organ trafficking and transplant tourism: A commentary on the global realities. American Journal of Transplantation [Internet]. 2008;**8**(5):925-929. Available from: https://pubmed.ncbi.nlm.nih.gov/18416734/

[57] Horvat LD, Shariff SZ, Garg AX. Global trends in the rates of living kidney donation. Kidney International [Internet]. 2009;**75**(10):1088-1098. Available from: https://pubmed.ncbi.nlm.nih.gov/19225540/

[58] Tan J, Mabood Khalil MA, Kee T, Tiong HY, Khan TT, El-Madhoun I, et al. Deceased donor kidney transplant policies in Asia – Implications on practice and recommendations for the future. The Lancet Regional Health - Southeast Asia [Internet]. 2024;**21**:1-10. Available from: http://www.thelancet.com/article/S2772368223001725/fulltext

[59] Watters TK, Glass BD, Mallett AJ. Identifying the barriers to kidney transplantation for patients in rural and remote areas: A scoping review. Journal of Nephrology [Internet]. 2023;**1**:1-13. Available from: https://link.springer.com/article/10.1007/s40620-023-01755-0

[60] Roberts LE, Kaur A, Jewitt-Harris J, Ready A, Milford DV. Kidney

transplantation in low- and middle-income countries: The transplant links experience. Pediatric Nephrology [Internet]. 2024;**39**(5):1347-1353. Available from: https://link.springer.com/article/10.1007/s00467-023-06129-z

[61] International Finance Corporation. Kyrgyz Republic: Dialysis centers PPP brief. International Finance Corporation. 2019. Available from: https://www.ifc.org/ppp

[62] Abuzaineh N, Brashers E, Foong S, Feachem R, Da Rita P. PPPs in healthcare: Models, lessons and trends for the future. Healthcare public-private partnership series, No. 4. The Global Health Group, Institute for Global Health Sciences, University of California, San Francisco, and PwC. 2018. Available from: https://tiny.ucsf.edu/globalhealthgroup

[63] Vincenti F, Rostaing L, Grinyo J, Rice K, Steinberg S, Gaite L, et al. Belatacept and long-term outcomes in kidney transplantation. New England Journal of Medicine [Internet]. 2016;**374**(4):333-343. DOI: 10.1056/NEJMoa1506027

[64] Neuen BL, Bello AK, Levin A, Lunney M, Osman MA, Ye F, et al. National health policies and strategies for addressing chronic kidney disease: Data from the International Society of Nephrology Global Kidney Health Atlas. PLOS Global Public Health [Internet]. 2023;**3**(2):e0001467. Available from: https://journals.plos.org/globalpublichealth/article?id=10.1371/journal.pgph.0001467

[65] Arshad A, Anderson B, Sharif A. Comparison of organ donation and transplantation rates between opt-out and opt-in systems. Kidney International [Internet]. 2019;**95**(6):1453-1460. Available from: https://pubmed.ncbi.nlm.nih.gov/31010718/ [Accessed: July 14, 2024]

[66] Luyckx VA, Al-Aly Z, Bello AK, Bellorin-Font E, Carlini RG, Fabian J, et al. Sustainable development goals relevant to kidney health: An update on progress. Nature Reviews. Nephrology [Internet]. 2021;**17**(1):15-32. Available from: https://pubmed.ncbi.nlm.nih.gov/33188362/ [Accessed: July 14, 2024]

[67] Patzer RE, Retzloff S, Buford J, Gander J, Browne T, Jones H, et al. Community engagement to improve equity in kidney transplantation from the ground up: The Southeastern kidney transplant coalition. Current Transplantation Reports [Internet]. 2021;**8**(4):324. Available from: /pmc/articles/PMC9435919/

[68] Kimmel PL, Jefferson N, Norton JM, Star RA. How community engagement is enhancing NIDDK research. Clinical Journal of the American Society of Nephrology [Internet]. 2019;**14**(5):768. Available from: /pmc/articles/PMC6500937/

[69] Aguilar-González A, Lou-Meda R, Chocó-Cedillos A, Moist L. Community engagement in kidney research: Guatemalan experience. BMC Nephrology [Internet]. 2022;**23**(1):1-9. Available from: https://bmcnephrol.biomedcentral.com/articles/10.1186/s12882-022-02891-8

[70] Concepcion BP, Forbes RC. The role of telemedicine in kidney transplantation: Opportunities and challenges. Kidney360 [Internet]. 2020;**1**(5):420. Available from: /pmc/articles/PMC8809293/

[71] Hezer B, Massey EK, Reinders MEJ, Tielen M, Van De Wetering J, Hesselink DA, et al. Telemedicine for kidney transplant recipients: Current state, advantages, and barriers. Transplantation [Internet]. 2024;**108**(2):409. Available from: /pmc/articles/PMC10798592/

[72] Duettmann W, Naik MG, Zukunft B, Osmonodja B, Bachmann F, Choi M, et al. eHealth in transplantation. Transplant International [Internet]. 2021;**34**(1):16-26. DOI: 10.1111/tri.13778

[73] Bellini A, Finocchietti M, Rosa AC, Nordio M, Ferroni E, Massari M, et al. Effectiveness and safety of immunosuppressive regimens used as maintenance therapy in kidney transplantation: The CESIT study. PLoS One [Internet]. 2024;**19**(1):e0295205. Available from: https://journals.plos.org/plosone/article?id=10.1371/journal.pone.0295205

[74] Hosgood SA, Brown RJ, Nicholson ML. Advances in kidney preservation techniques and their application in clinical practice. Transplantation [Internet]. 2021;**105**(11):e202. Available from: /pmc/articles/PMC8549459/

[75] Drain PK, Hyle EP, Noubary F, Freedberg KA, Wilson D, Bishai WR, et al. Diagnostic point-of-care tests in resource-limited settings. The Lancet Infectious Diseases [Internet]. 2014;**14**(3):239-249. Available from: http://www.thelancet.com/article/S1473309913702500/fulltext

[76] Yager P, Domingo GJ, Gerdes J. Point-of-care diagnostics for global health. Annual Review of Biomedical Engineering. 2008;**10**:107-144. DOI: 10.1146/annurev.bioeng.10.061807.160524

[77] Fan K, Zhao Y. Mobile health technology: A novel tool in chronic disease management. Intelligent Medicine. 2022;**2**(1):41-47

[78] Zan S, Agboola S, Moore SA, Parks KA, Kvedar JC, Jethwani K. Patient engagement with a mobile web-based telemonitoring system for heart failure self-management: A pilot study. JMIR mHealth and uHealth [Internet]. 2015;**3**(2):e33. Available from: http://www.ncbi.nlm.nih.gov/pubmed/25842282

[79] José Medina Pestana A, Medina PJ. Clinical outcomes of 11,436 kidney transplants performed in a single center - Hospital do Rim. Brazilian. Journal of Nephrology. 2017;**39**(3):287-295. Available from: https://www.scielo.br/j/jbn/a/VsVwSqpRmLGHjg8fphmNn4J/?lang=en

[80] Medina-Pestana JO. Organization of a high-volume kidney transplant program - the “assembly line” approach. Transplantation [Internet]. 2006;**81**(11):1510-1520. Available from: https://journals.lww.com/transplantjournal/fulltext/2006/06150/organization_of_a_high_volume_kidney_transplant.3.aspx

[81] Groote Schuur Hospital Transplants 30th Kidney This Year – Western Cape Government [Internet]. Available from: https://www.westerncape.gov.za/news/groote-schuur-hospital-transplants-30th-kidney-year

Chapter 2

Recurrent Focal Segmental Glomerulosclerosis Post Renal Transplantation

Maiko Alejandro Tavera Díaz, David Andrés Ballesteros Castro, Omar Lafuente Covarrubias, Alison Vannia Nava Rojas and Israel Danny Rivas Salazar

Abstract

Focal segmental glomerulosclerosis (FSGS) is a major cause of nephrotic syndrome in children and adults, presenting a significant clinical challenge due to its high post-transplant recurrence rate and its negative impact on graft survival. The pathophysiology of recurrent FSGS (rFSGS) involves a complex interplay between circulating permeability factors and podocyte signaling pathways, leading to actin cytoskeleton disorganization and glomerular filtration barrier dysfunction. This review explores the epidemiology, risk factors, and pathogenic mechanisms of rFSGS, focusing on the central role of podocytes and their intricate molecular architecture. Emerging biomarkers and potential therapeutic strategies are also discussed, based on our current understanding of the disease. Further studies are needed to fully elucidate the precise mechanisms and develop targeted therapies to improve outcomes in patients with post-transplant rFSGS.

Keywords: FSGS, kidney transplantation, recurrence, podocytes, proteinuria

1. Introduction

FSGS is a clinicopathological syndrome manifesting with proteinuria, typically in the nephrotic range, originating from histopathological findings of hyalinosis, sclerosis, foot process effacement (FPE), and glomerular scarring that progresses to generalized glomerulosclerosis in advanced stages [1]. Nephrotic syndrome (NS) in 20% of children and 40% of adults originates from FSGS. The annual incidence ranges from 0.2 to 2.5 cases per 100,000 population, varying by race and age, accounting for about 4% of end-stage kidney disease (ESKD) causes, with progression rates to ESKD as high as 30–50% within 5–10 years post-diagnosis [2–4].

FSGS is classified etiologically into the following:

1. Primary, attributed to "permeability factors" or "circulating factors" causing podocyte dysfunction.

2. Familial or genetic, due to mutations in molecules composing the basal-apical domain and slit diaphragm.

3. Secondary to viral infections, drugs, adaptive structural-functional responses.

4. Indeterminate, when a clear etiology is not identified [5].

Post-transplant rFSGS is defined as the appearance of nephrotic proteinuria and hypoalbuminemia in a patient with a history of primary FSGS in their native kidneys, along with characteristic histological findings of FSGS in the renal allograft biopsy [6].

2. Podocyte physiology

Podocytes are mesoderm-derived cells, 5–10 microns in diameter, with a complex cellular organization and cytoskeleton. They are composed of four segments: the cell body, primary processes, ridge-like prominence, and foot processes (FPE) [7]. Primary processes originate from the cell body, and FPEs branch from the ridge-like prominence of the basal portion of the cell body and primary process, visualized by transmission electron microscopy (TEM) of serial ultrathin sections and reconstruction. The ridge-like prominence of the primary processes serves as an adhesion medium to the basement membrane [7].

2.1 Functional domains of podocytes, etc.

2.1.1 Basal domain

This domain directly contacts the glomerular basement membrane (GBM). FPE adhesion to the GBM occurs via cell adhesion proteins called integrins, which are extracellular matrix receptors that connect the actin cytoskeleton through focal adhesions. Detailed descriptions of each protein and its interaction with actin are provided (**Figure 1**).

Integrin $\alpha3\beta1$: These receptors bind various extracellular matrix components such as laminin, collagen, or arginine-glycine-aspartic acid. Laminin-521 binding to integrin $\alpha3\beta1$ on the GBM induces a conformational change in the integrin, recruiting adapter proteins like talin, paxillin, and vinculin, which in turn recruit focal adhesion kinase (FAK) and integrin-linked kinase (ILK) to form a mature focal adhesion complex, initiating signaling pathways: (1) FAK autophosphorylates and activates downstream signaling pathways like PI3K/Akt and Ras/MAPK that regulate cell survival, proliferation, and motility. (2) ILK interacts with nephrin, regulating its phosphorylation and function. (3) Small GTPases activated by integrin signaling pathways regulate actin cytoskeleton dynamics in podocytes. RhoA promotes stress fiber formation and focal adhesions, while Rac1 and Cdc42 promote lamellipodia and

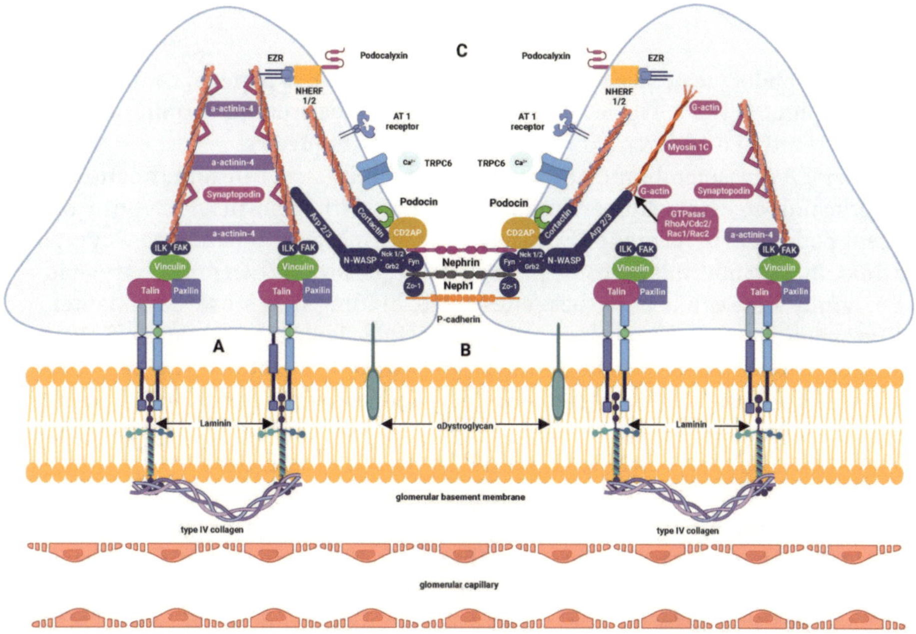

Figure 1.
Podocyte physiology: Integrin α3β1 binds laminin-521 on GBM, inducing integrin clustering and focal adhesion complex formation. Talin binds integrin β1 subunit's cytoplasmic domain, activating integrin, recruiting adapter proteins and cytoskeleton regulators like vinculin, stabilizing focal adhesions, and reinforcing actin cytoskeleton connection. α-Actinin-4 bundles actin filaments, anchoring them to focal adhesions via vinculin and talin interactions. Paxillin phosphorylates in response to cell adhesion and mechanical tension, creating binding sites for signaling and adapter proteins regulating focal adhesion dynamics and actin cytoskeleton reorganization. Nephrin and Neph1 interact via extracellular domains, forming SD scaffold. Their cytoplasmic domains bind CD2AP and ZO-1, acting as adapter proteins interacting with cortactin and α-actinin-4, respectively, linking to actin. Nephrin's phosphorylated tyrosine sites bind Nck, recruiting adapter proteins like N-WASP, activating Arp2/3 complex, and promoting actin polymerization and branching. Podocin interacts with nephrin and Neph1 cytoplasmic domains, stabilizing SD complex. Podocalyxin and podoendin are located on podocyte apical plasma membrane with extracellular domains facing the urinary space. Their cytoplasmic domains interact with NHERF2's PDZ domain and ezrin's FERM domain, forming a PODXL-NHERF2-ezrin complex. Ezrin's C-terminal domain binds actin filaments in its active (T567-phosphorylated) conformation. These interactions connect podocalyxin and ezrin to underlying actin cytoskeleton.

filopodia formation, respectively. Balanced activation of these GTPases is essential for maintaining podocyte morphology and function [8].

Integrin αvβ3: Composed of two non-covalently associated subunits (αv and β3), each with a large extracellular domain, a single transmembrane domain, and a short cytoplasmic tail. Integrin αvβ3 interacts with cytoplasmic proteins like talin, kindlin, paxillin, and FAK, important for αvβ3-mediated signaling and its connection to the actin cytoskeleton. In podocytes, αvβ3 mediates adhesion to the GBM and may regulate the architecture and function of podocyte processes, contributing to GBM adhesion and podocyte function regulation [9].

α-Dystroglycan: A highly glycosylated extracellular protein binding to GBM components like laminin, agrin, and perlecan. β-Dystroglycan, a transmembrane protein, connects intracellularly with cytoskeletal proteins like utrophin [8]. In podocytes, the dystroglycan complex acts as a molecular bridge between the GBM and intracellular actin cytoskeleton, crucial for proper podocyte-GBM anchoring and maintaining podocyte process structure.

2.1.2 Lateral domain

Adjacent podocyte pedicels interdigitate in a zipper-like pattern, connected by the slit diaphragm (SD). The SD is composed of various proteins forming a molecular sieve contributing to glomerular filtration function (**Figure 1**).

Nephrin: A transmembrane protein essential for SD structure and function. It has three domains: an extracellular domain interacting with nephrin and neph1 from adjacent podocytes to form the SD, a short transmembrane domain, and a cytoplasmic domain with multiple tyrosine phosphorylation sites. When phosphorylated by Src family kinases like Fyn, these sites create binding sites for several adapter and signaling proteins, allowing nephrin to scaffold signaling complexes [8, 10]. Phosphorylated tyrosines can be divided into two groups: group A (Y1114, Y1138/9) recruiting p85/PI3K, activating Akt and Rac1, and leading to cofilin activation regulating actin dynamics; group B (Y1176, Y1193, and Y1217) recruits adapter proteins Nck and Grb2. Nck recruits N-WASp and PAK; N-WASp activates the Arp2/3 complex nucleating new actin filaments, promoting actin polymerization and branching. PAK also regulates the actin cytoskeleton by phosphorylating downstream substrates [10]. Nephrin phosphorylation and these signaling factors' recruitment lead to localized actin remodeling, maintaining podocyte process architecture. Phosphatases like SHP-1 and PTP1B can dephosphorylate nephrin, providing negative control of this signaling pathway. Altered nephrin phosphorylation and actin signaling are implicated in podocyte diseases characterized by process loss and proteinuria [10]. Nephrin also interacts with adapter protein CD2AP, directly binding actin and stabilizing the actin cytoskeleton in podocyte processes [8].

Neph1: A transmembrane protein structurally similar to nephrin, forming heterodimers with nephrin via extracellular interactions, essential for SD formation and maintenance. Neph1's cytoplasmic domain has tyrosine phosphorylation sites similar to nephrin, recruiting adapter protein Grb2 upon phosphorylation and aiding actin polymerization [8, 11]. Neph1 also interacts with podocin and adapter proteins like ZO-1, binding actin and stabilizing the actin cytoskeleton [8, 11].

Podocin: A hairpin-like protein with N- and C-terminal cytoplasmic domains located in lipid rafts, stabilizing nephrin at the SD. Podocin interacts with Neph1, CD2AP, and indirectly connects the SD complex with the actin cytoskeleton [8, 11, 12].

CD2AP: A cytoplasmic adapter protein linking nephrin and podocin through its N-terminal domain and interacting with actin via cortactin. CD2AP acts as a molecular scaffold stabilizing SD structure and anchoring it to the actin cytoskeleton [8, 11, 12].

ZO-1: An adapter protein at tight junctions and SD in podocytes. ZO-1 binds Neph1's cytoplasmic domain, scaffolding SD complex to actin cytoskeleton. ZO-1 also interacts with actin-regulating proteins like α-actinin-4, organizing and stabilizing actin filaments in pedicels [8, 11].

P-Cadherin: A transmembrane SD protein co-localizing with ZO-1, forming links with F-actin [11].

TRPC6: A non-selective cation channel interacting with nephrin and podocin, allowing intracellular $Ca2+$ influx, increasing cytosolic calcium in response to mechanical stress and angiotensin II, activating calcineurin signaling pathways, a calcium-dependent phosphatase dephosphorylating and degrading synaptopodin, altering actin filament stability, and compromising podocyte structural integrity [8, 11, 12].

Synaptopodin: A cytoplasmic protein binding actin filaments, positively regulating RhoA activity, and stabilizing actin by protecting from cofilin action, an actin-severing and disassembling protein. Synaptopodin interacts with α-actinin-4, directly with TRPC6, regulating its localization and activity in podocyte plasma membrane. Under stress or injury, synaptopodin is phosphorylated by PKA and CaMKII, increasing its stability and actin filament stabilization capacity [12].

α-Actinin-4: A protein cross-linking actin filaments in a scaffold-like manner in actin cytoskeleton assembly, interacting with GBM via integrins [8, 11, 12].

2.1.3 Actin cytoskeleton

F-actin is localized in submembranous regions of podocyte membrane domains. GBM is connected to this actin network by dystroglycan, integrins, and focal adhesion complex molecules like talin, paxillin, and vinculin. At SD, nephrin/podocin complex binding is mediated by CD2AP. P-cadherin may use ZO-1 for this purpose. Finally, at the apical membrane domain, NHERV-2 and ezrin indirectly link podocalyxin to actin (**Figure 1**) [12].

Actin Structure in Podocytes: Podocytes contain 42 kDa globular actin (G-actin) monomers assembling into polarized actin filaments (F-actin). In podocyte processes, actin filaments organize into two main structures: a central bundle of loosely packed actin filaments along the process's longitudinal axis and a cortical actin network associated with cortactin surrounding the central bundle [13]. The polymerization process, forming actin filaments, begins with small GTPases like RhoA, Rac1, and Cdc42 activation. These GTPases are regulated by GAP (GTPase-activating proteins), GEF (guanine nucleotide exchange factors), and GDI (guanine nucleotide dissociation inhibitors) proteins [13, 14]. Once activated, GTPases interact with specific effectors to regulate actin dynamics. RhoA interacts with formin, and Rac1 and Cdc42 activate N-WASP and Arp2/3, inducing nucleation, forming a three-actin-G monomer nucleus, leading to a branched actin filament network. After nucleation, G-actin monomers add to growing F-actin ends. Once formed, F-actin filaments cross-link and bundle by α-actinin-4 and non-muscle myosins (Myo1e), forming bundles and networks (**Figure 1**) [13, 14]. Increased RhoA and decreased Rac1/Cdc42 generate stationary podocytes with intact processes; the reverse promotes motility and podocyte effacement. Balancing RhoA activity against Rac/Cdc42 is crucial for actin cytoskeleton maintenance [13, 14].

Proteins like profilin facilitate ADP-ATP exchange in actin monomers, promoting addition to growing filaments. Others, like Ena/VASP, bind filament ends, promoting elongation by preventing capping proteins [13, 14]. Actin filament depolymerization is regulated by proteins like cofilin and gelsolin. Cofilin binds actin filaments, promoting fragmentation and G-actin monomer dissociation. Cofilin activity is regulated by phosphorylation: LIMK phosphorylation inactivates cofilin, while phosphatases like slingshot activate it [13, 14]. Gelsolin is a capping protein binding filament ends, preventing elongation and promoting depolymerization [13, 14].

2.1.4 Apical domain

Facing the urinary space, containing proteins interacting with actin cytoskeleton, contributing to podocyte function and integrity. Each protein's detailed description and actin interaction are provided (**Figure 1**) [8, 11].

Podocalyxin (PODXL): A heavily negatively charged sialomucin abundantly expressed on podocyte apical surface, interacting with actin cytoskeleton. Podocalyxin's cytoplasmic domain contains ERM-binding and NHERF-binding domains. Through these domains, podocalyxin recruits ezrin and NHERF2, interacting with actin and regulating actin cytoskeleton organization in pedicels [8, 11].

Ezrin: A member of the ERM protein family, linking the apical plasma membrane and actin cytoskeleton. Ezrin has two conformations: inactive folded and active unfolded. Ezrin phosphorylation at T567 by PKC and ROCK activates it. In active conformation, ezrin binds podocalyxin's ERM-binding domain via its N-terminal FERM domain and actin filaments via its C-terminal domain. Connecting podocalyxin to actin cytoskeleton, ezrin helps maintain pedicel morphology and podocalyxin distribution on the apical surface [8, 11].

NHERF2: An adapter protein with two PDZ domains and an ERM-binding domain. NHERF2 binds podocalyxin via PDZ domain and ezrin via ERM domain, forming a ternary PODXL-NHERF2-ezrin complex. This complex is crucial for maintaining pedicel structure and function, regulating podocyte cell signaling [8, 11].

Podoendin: A transmembrane glycoprotein expressed on podocyte apical surface. Although its exact function is not fully understood, podoendin may regulate pedicel morphology and cell signaling in podocytes. Podoendin's cytoplasmic domain contains a PDZ-binding motif, interacting with PDZ domain-containing adapter proteins like NHERF2, indirectly connecting to actin cytoskeleton, contributing to pedicel organization [8, 11].

3. Epidemiology

3.1 Incidence

rFSGS epidemiology post-kidney transplant varies by patient age and race. Incidence ranges from 6 to 60%, depending on the studies reviewed [6].

A meta-analysis found higher rFSGS cumulative incidence in the first renal transplant in children (50–60%) compared to adults (20–40%) [15]. rFSGS incidence in the second renal transplant is around 80% [16]. By race, a review shows rFSGS is more common in patients of European ancestry than non-European. In Caucasians, the cumulative incidence is 27.98% (range: 17.27–40.14%) and in non-Caucasians, it is 14.0% (range: 12.2–15.9%) [16]. In a US cohort study, FSGS recurrence rate was 27% in Caucasian transplant recipients [17]. A US registry analysis found non-Caucasian transplant recipients had a significantly lower risk of FSGS recurrence compared to Caucasians (HR 0.45; 95% CI: 0.28–0.72) [18]. In a US pediatric study, FSGS recurrence rate was 29% in African American recipients compared to 50% in Caucasians [19]. Another US study reported a 27% recurrence rate in adult African Americans [20]. For Asian race, a Korean study found a 30% recurrence rate after renal transplant in a pediatric cohort [21]. A Japanese study found a 25% recurrence rate in pediatric patients [22]. Limited data are available for Hispanic/Latino incidence; a US study reported a 50% recurrence rate in Hispanic transplant recipients (**Table 1**) [20].

3.2 Kidney graft survival in rFSGS

A retrospective analysis of the North American Pediatric Renal Transplant Cooperative Study (NAPRTCS) database, including 6484 children who received

Age/race	Caucasian	African American	Asian	Hispanic/Latino
Children	50% [19]	29% [19]	30% [21]	N/A
			25% [22]	
Adults	27% [17], 38% [20]	27% [20]	N/A	50% [20]

N/A: no specific data available in the mentioned studies.

Table 1.
Epidemiology of focal and segmental glomerulosclerosis post kidney transplantation.

kidney transplants, with 752 (11.6%) diagnosed with FSGS. Graft survival was significantly worse in FSGS patients who received transplants from living donors (LD). The 5-year graft survival rate was 69% in FSGS patients compared to 82% in non-FSGS patients [22]. Another retrospective cohort study of 1505 kidney transplant patients found graft loss due to rFSGS at 10 years was 8.4%, higher than acute rejection incidence (4.1%). Graft loss incidence due to recurrence was significantly higher in FSGS recipients (adjusted hazard ratio 2.03) [23]. A meta-analysis of 22 studies with 966 patients, 358 with recurrent FSGS and 608 without post-transplant FSGS, found recurrent FSGS patients had a 52% graft survival rate at 5 years compared to 83% in non-recurrent FSGS patients. The 5-year graft survival was significantly higher in non-rFSGS patients (OR 4.24; 95% CI 2.77–6.48; $P < 0.001$). This recurrence significantly impacts graft survival [24].

4. Pathogenesis of FSGS recurrence

4.1 T and B lymphocyte dysfunction

FSGS is a challenging renal disease studied for decades. The "Shalhoub Theory" proposed over 50 years ago laid the foundation for investigating T-lymphocyte dysfunction and permeability factor release as potential causes of podocyte damage [25]. Numerous studies have highlighted the fundamental role of T and B lymphocytes in idiopathic nephrotic syndrome (INS) pathogenesis, including FSGS. Two independent studies demonstrated clonal expansions of predominantly CD8+ T lymphocytes in complicated INS patients [26, 27]. These expansions, identified by CDR3 (complementarity-determining region 3) diversity analysis of the T-cell receptor (TCR) β-chain, were more frequent and persistent in patients with frequent relapses or FSGS compared to infrequent relapses [26, 27]. These findings suggest that clonally expanded cytotoxic T cells could be a key factor in disease progression. Immunophenotypic alterations in different NS types, including corticosteroid-dependent/frequent relapse nephrotic syndrome (SDNS/FRNS), MCD, and FSGS. Findings highlight T- and B-cell interactions' importance in these diseases' pathogenesis, suggesting potential biomarkers for predicting rituximab treatment response [28]. In adult SDNS/FRNS patients, a significant reduction in FOXP3+ regulatory T cells (Tregs), especially CD45RO+ memory Tregs, was observed compared to corticosteroid-resistant nephrotic syndrome (SRNS) patients and healthy volunteers [28]. Additionally, baseline memory Treg levels were significantly lower in patients relapsing after rituximab treatment [28]. These findings suggest Treg deficiency, particularly memory Tregs, may contribute to corticosteroid dependence and frequent relapses in SDNS/FRNS, with baseline memory Treg levels potentially serving as a rituximab response biomarker [28]. Relapses were associated with increased specific T cell subpopulations, including increased CD4 + CD45RO + CXCR5+ (memory T) cells and decreased Tregs (CD4 + CD25highFoxP3high) and IL2 expression [29]. In FSGS patients, relapses were characterized by increased activated T- and B-cell populations, including helper T cells (CD4+), cytotoxic T cells (CD8+), memory T cells (CD45RO+), and memory B cells (CD27+ IgD-/IgM-) [30]. These findings align with previous MCNS and FSGS studies, suggesting activated T and B cell alterations are a hallmark of these diseases [30]. In addition to CD8+ T cell alterations, increased circulating T helper 17 (Th17) cells were observed in INS patients, more pronounced in FSGS than MCD. Th17 cells produce interleukin-17 (IL-17), a proinflammatory cytokine with deleterious effects on podocytes through Fas/Caspase-8/Caspase-3 pathway activation. Elevated IL-17 and IL-1β levels were found in FSGS patients' renal tissue [31]. In relapsing steroid-sensitive nephrotic syndrome (SSNS) children, a significant increase in memory IgM B cells (CD27 + IgD + IgM+) and switched memory B cells (CD27 + IgD-IgM-) with notable decrease in transitional B cells (CD19 + CD24hiCD38hi) was observed [32]. A study demonstrated a 20.5% transitional B-cell cutoff value (as a percentage of total lymphocytes) differentiating SSNS from SRNS with 79.1% sensitivity and 90.9% specificity [32]. These findings suggest lower transitional B-cell proportion and higher memory B-cell proportion as relapse risk indicators in SRNS patients. Treg and Breg deficiencies, increased activated T and B cells appear common in SDNS/FRNS, MCNS, and FSGS, with specific subpopulation differences [28, 30, 33]. Rituximab treatment seems to modulate these immunological alterations, leading to remission in many patients. However, further studies are needed to elucidate rituximab's exact therapeutic mechanisms and validate potential biomarkers identified in these studies [28, 30]. Another study identified elevated plasmablasts (CD24 - CD38 hi CD27 hi) correlated with increased IL-21, IL-6, and B-cell activating factor (BAFF) cytokines and proteinuria [34]. BAFF promotes peripheral B-cell viability, development, and differentiation into plasma cells. Excessive BAFF stimulation bypasses and counteracts immature B-cell negative selection or death signals, creating survival signals for autoreactive B cells, losing B-cell tolerance, and developing autoimmune diseases [35]. These studies provide new insights into T- and B-cell roles in FSGS pathogenesis, suggesting potential rituximab treatment biomarkers [28, 30]. However, further research is needed to translate these findings into clinical applications and develop more specific therapeutic approaches addressing underlying immunological alterations in this disease [28, 30].

4.2 Monocyte dysfunction

The "monocyte activation theory" is attractive because monocyte activation could originate T- and B-cell dysfunction, altered cytokine, and antibody production. Monocytes are fundamental for innate and adaptive immunity due to their differentiation capability into specialized cells, enabling highly adaptable immune responses. These cells play a crucial role in stimulating B-cell proliferation and differentiation. Interferon gamma (IFN-γ) and interleukin 10 (IL-10) induce BAFF release in monocytes, essential for B-cell survival and maturation, negatively regulated by IL-4. Monocytes increase BAFF and soluble urokinase plasminogen activator receptor (sUPAR), contributing to B-cell activation. These mechanisms are implicated in FSGS pathogenesis [35]. Monocytes express CD40 receptors on their surface, allowing activation by sCD40L released by activated CD4 lymphocytes. Activated monocytes respond to sCD40L and produce and release it, creating a positive feedback loop.

This activation increases proinflammatory cytokine production like TNF-α, IL-1β, and IL-6, adhesion molecule expression, reactive oxygen species production, and monocyte differentiation into macrophages. The sCD40L-monocyte interaction plays a crucial role in inflammatory processes, promoting more inflammatory cell recruitment. In renal diseases like FSGS, this interaction could significantly contribute to pathogenesis, where chronic monocyte activation and sustained sCD40L production could exacerbate renal damage [36, 37]. A single-cell RNA-seq study of urine from FSGS patients identified two main monocyte subtypes: M1 and M2. M1 monocytes expressed proinflammatory genes like IL1B and CCL2, suggesting they contribute to renal inflammation by recruiting and activating other immune cells. These cells initiate and maintain adaptive immune responses like T-cell activation. In FSGS, these monocytes could bridge innate and adaptive immunity, amplifying and perpetuating renal inflammation [38].

4.3 Permeability factors

Identifying a circulating permeability factor in pFSGS patients' blood has been a long-standing interest and debate, identifying several potential agents responsible for podocyte dysfunction **Figure 2** [64]. In the 1990s, Savin et al. conducted an in vitro study isolating rat glomeruli incubated with sera from rFSGS patients, generating

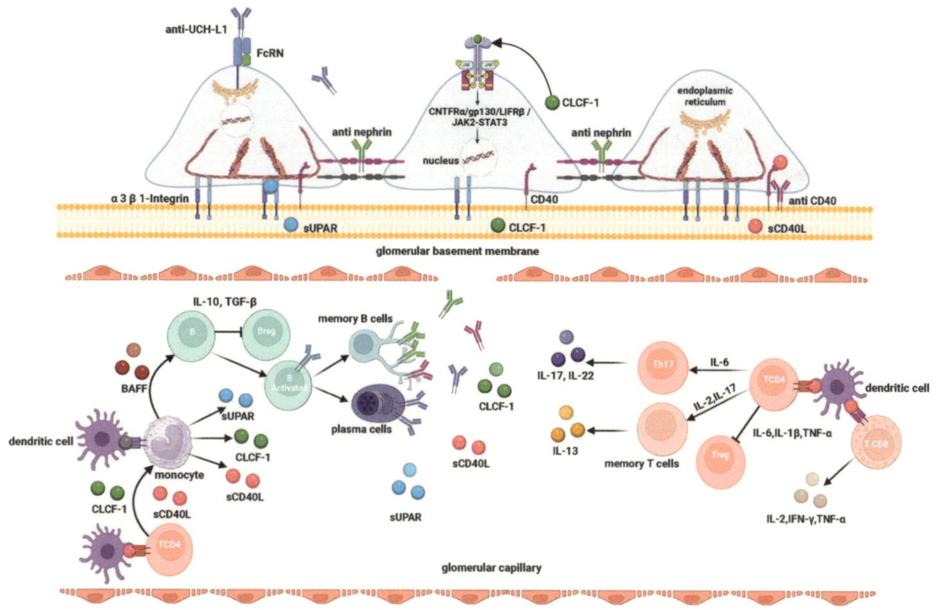

Figure 2.
*Anti-nephrin antibody: inhibits nephrin, compromising slit diaphragm function and causing proteinuria. Anti-UCH-L1 antibody: alters protein homeostasis in podocytes, contributing to dysfunction and cell death. Anti-CD40 antibody: activates inflammatory pathways binding to CD40, contributing to podocyte damage and dysfunction. sCD40L: binds CD40 on podocytes, inducing inflammation and autoimmune responses resulting in podocyte damage. CLCF-1: activates JAK2-STAT3 pathway, contributing to inflammation and structural damage in podocytes. suPAR: binds αvβ3 integrin, inducing podocyte activation and cytoskeleton rearrangement causing proteinuria and podocyte damage. Hemopexin: associated with inflammation and renal damage, exact mechanism unclear. IL-13: induces extracellular matrix protein expression changes, contributing to inflammation and renal fibrosis. TNF-α: induces podocyte apoptosis and damage, resulting in inflammation and filtration barrier dysfunction. BAFF: promotes B-cell survival and activation, contributing to autoantibody production and immune damage in podocytes (**Table** 2).*

Permeability factor	Origin	Molecular weight	Mechanism of podocyte injury	Treatment
Anti-nephrin antibodies [39, 40]	Autoreactive B cells	~150 kDa (IgG)	Binding nephrin induces tyrosine phosphorylation and cytoskeletal alterations	B-cell depletion therapy (rituximab) and plasmapheresis
Anti-UCH-L1 antibodies [41, 42]	Autoreactive B cells	~150 kDa (IgG)	Induces podocyte apoptosis and alters intracellular UCH-L1 concentration	Corticosteroids (steroid-sensitive), rituximab (steroid-resistant), and plasmapheresis
Anti-CD40 antibodies [43, 44]	Autoreactive B cells	~150 kDa (IgG)	Binding CD40 prolongs suPAR-mediated integrin activation	B-cell depletion therapy (rituximab) and plasmapheresis
CLCF-1 [45–47]	Activated T cells, various tissues	22 kDa	JAK2/STAT3 pathway activation and cytoskeletal alterations	JAK2 or STAT3 inhibitors, oral galactose therapy (contradictory)
SuPAR [48–51]	Activated immune cells	55–60 kDa	$\alpha v \beta 3$ integrin signaling activation and foot process effacement	No specific treatment established
Hemopexin [52–54]	Liver, glomerular mesangial cells	60 kDa	Nephrin-dependent actin reorganization and podocyte damage	No specific treatment established
Interleukin-13 (IL-13) [55–57]	Produced by Th2, CD4+ and CD8+ T cells	12–13 kDa	1. Decreased transepithelial electrical resistance in cultured podocytes 2. Reduced glomerular expression of nephrin, podocin, and dystroglycan 3. Increased glomerular expression of B7-1 (CD80) 4. Destabilization of the slit diaphragm 5. Direct effect on podocytes through IL-13 receptors	Potential therapeutic strategies: 1. Blocking IL-13 2. Inhibition of IL-13 signaling pathways Note: clinical studies are needed to validate these approaches
TNF-α [58, 59]	Various immune cells	17 kDa (soluble), 26 kDa (transmembrane)	TNF signaling pathway activation and upregulation of TNF-α expression	Anti-TNF-α monoclonal antibodies (adalimumab)
BAFF [60–63]	Monocytes, T cells, neutrophils, dendritic cells	31–35 kDa	Autoreactive B-cell survival and autoantibody production	Belimumab (lupus nephritis, efficacy in FSGS not established)

Table 2.
Characteristics of permeability factors.

increased glomerular albumin permeability (Palbumin) above 0.50, and predicting recurrence with 60% sensitivity and 95% specificity [16]. Gallon et al. published a case report of a pFSGS recipient receiving a related living donor transplant, developing proteinuria on the second post-transplant day. After ethics committee approval, the graft was removed and re-implanted in another ESKD recipient secondary to diabetic renal disease, with subsequent normal renal function and proteinuria. This pioneering decision confirms the presence of an extrarenal permeability factor [65]. The following reviews potential permeability factors responsible for rFSGS: **Figure 2** and **Table 3**.

Autoantibodies: Autoantibodies targeting podocyte antigens produced by autoreactive B cells have emerged as potential mediators of podocyte damage in FSGS and other podocytopathies.

Anti-nephrin antibodies: Anti-nephrin antibodies are IgG immunoglobulins produced by autoreactive B cells. Binding to nephrin induces nephrin tyrosine phosphorylation, triggering actin cytoskeleton alterations characterized by foot process effacement and basal parallel actin filament attenuation [66]. A multicenter

Immune cells	Dysfunction/implications in FSGS	Cytokines/production factors
T lymphocytes		
• CD4+ (T helper) [27]	Clonal expansion of CD8+ T cells and Th17 in FSGS	IL-2, IL-4, IL-5, and IL-21
• CD8+ (cytotoxic T) [27]	Clonal expansion in patients with frequent relapses	IFN-γ
• Treg (regulatory) [28, 29]	Decreased in SDNS/FRNS, especially memory Tregs	IL-10 and TGF-β
• Memory T cells [30]	Increased in FSGS and related pathologies	Various cytokines depending on subgroup
• Th17 [31]	Increased in FSGS, podocyte damage via Fas/caspase pathway	IL-17 and IL-22
B lymphocytes		
• Mature B cells [30, 32]	Increased in relapses	Specific antibodies
• Memory B cells	Increased in relapses	Specific antibodies
• Transitional B [32]	Decreased in SSNS/SRNS, correlated with relapse risk	—
• Plasma cells [34]	Elevated plasmablasts correlated with cytokines like IL-21, IL-6, and BAFF	Specific antibodies
Monocytes		
• M1 [35–38]	Contribute to renal inflammation and activation of other immune cells	IL-1β, TNF-α, IL-6, and CCL2
• M2 [38]	Anti-inflammatory and profibrotic action	IL-10 and TGF-β
• General [35–38]	Involved in B-cell activation and pro-inflammatory cytokine production	sUPAR, BAFF, sCD40L, and CLCF-1

Table 3.
Immune system dysfunction.

observational study of 22 pediatric FSGS patients (11 primary and 8 genetic) revealed significant findings. Primary FSGS patients had significantly elevated anti-nephrin antibody levels (average 899 U/ml and normal <231 U/ml). Histology showed IgG deposits colocalized with nephrin, mainly IgG3 and IgG4 subclasses, and C3 deposits not colocalizing with nephrin. Increased phosphorylated nephrin and Src/ShcA (collagen-A) expression, along with altered nephrin and FPE distribution, were observed. These findings were not seen in genetic FSGS, other glomerulonephritides, or healthy controls [67]. Recently, Hengel et al. published an observational study showing a high prevalence of anti-nephrin antibodies in various populations. In children with active INS and nephrotic-range proteinuria, prevalence was 90%. In adults, 44% of MCD cases and 9% of FSGS cases had these antibodies. Their presence strongly correlated with MCD activity and nephrotic-range proteinuria pre-treatment. Additionally, 38% of relapsing MCD cases had these antibodies. In contrast, prevalence was significantly lower in other glomerulonephritides and healthy controls [39, 40]. These findings underscore anti-nephrin antibodies' importance in certain nephrotic syndrome forms' pathogenesis and diagnosis, offering new insights into understanding and managing these renal diseases.

Anti-ubiquitin C-terminal hydrolase L1 (anti-UCH-L1) antibodies: UCH-L1 is a deubiquitinating enzyme removing ubiquitins from proteins marked for degradation, crucial for intracellular protein quality control. Dysfunctional UCH-L1 generates ubiquitinated protein accumulation, contributing to podocyte injury [68]. UCH-L1 receptors are expressed on podocyte surfaces and interiors, especially endoplasmic reticulum and nucleus. Circulating anti-UCH-L1 autoantibodies bind UCH-L1 on podocyte apical domains, forming in situ immune complexes, internalized via neonatal Fc receptor (FcRn)-mediated transcytosis. These immune complexes alter signaling pathways affecting actin cytoskeleton organization in podocytes [68, 69]. A basic and translational research study combining in vitro experiments, proteomic analyses, and an animal model investigated autoantibodies' role in INS. The study began with the discovery that plasma fractions containing IgG from relapsing INS patients, but not from controls or patients in remission, induced cultured human podocyte detachment. This suggested specific podocyte autoantibodies in active INS patients. Proteomic analyses identified UCH-L1 as a key podocyte autoantigen recognized by relapsing INS patients' IgG [69]. Further experiments showed UCH-L1 is expressed on podocyte surfaces and interiors, and commercial anti-UCH-L1 antibodies induced cultured podocyte detachment. Plasma IgG anti-UCH-L1 levels were significantly elevated in relapsing INS patients compared to controls and patients in remission, correlating with proteinuria at different disease stages [69]. To validate anti-UCH-L1 autoantibodies' causal role in INS, researchers injected purified patient anti-UCH-L1 IgG into mice, causing significant proteinuria and podocyte foot process effacement, mirroring key INS characteristics [41].

Soluble CD40 ligand (sCD40L) and anti-CD40 antibodies: CD40, a transmembrane glycoprotein in the TNF receptor superfamily, is expressed on podocyte basal domains in pathological conditions. sCD40L is released by T lymphocytes and monocytes, binding podocyte CD40, triggering damage mechanisms: (1) nephrin redistribution signaling pathway activation; (2) suPAR-mediated integrin ($\alpha v\beta 3$) activation and signaling pathway activation altering actin cytoskeleton organization; (3) matrix metalloproteinase (MMP) production induction degrading extracellular matrix contributing to glomerular damage; (4) podocyte apoptosis induction [42, 70]. Recent translational research sheds new light on CD40/CD40L system and related antibodies in primary podocytopathies' pathogenesis, specifically FSGS. A study combining in vitro, in vivo, and clinical analyses of 96 nephrotic syndrome patients and 11 healthy controls showed sCD40L rapidly reduces nephrin expression, reorganizes the cytoskeleton, and increases glomerular albumin permeability. These effects were blocked by CD40-CD40L interaction inhibitors. Clinically, elevated sCD40L serum levels were observed in nephrotic syndrome patients, with sCD40L detected in plasma fractions of post-transplant FSGS recurrence patients [37]. Another cross-sectional observational study of 106 glomerulopathy patients evaluated anti-CD40 and anti-UCH-L1 antibody levels. Results revealed elevated anti-UCH-L1 antibody levels in MCD and steroid-sensitive FSGS patients, suggesting potential as a good prognosis marker. In contrast, high anti-CD40 antibody levels were associated with steroid-resistant FSGS, indicating potential as a poor therapeutic response marker [43]. sCD40L seems to directly damage podocytes, while anti-CD40 and anti-UCH-L1 antibodies could serve as prognostic biomarkers. CD40 expressed on damaged podocytes serves as a target for anti-CD40 antibodies, enhancing suPAR-mediated integrin activation, increasing podocyte motility and loss [43, 70]. Anti-CD40 antibodies might play a crucial role, likely formed by autoreactive B lymphocytes due to factors like immunological tolerance loss, abnormal CD40 exposure on damaged podocytes acting as an antigen triggering an immune response, or molecular mimicry where some infections produce CD40-like proteins leading to cross-reactivity [42, 44]. An innovative in vitro study revealed anti-CD40 and suPAR antibodies' crucial role in FSGS. Using immortalized human podocytes and samples from recurrent and non-recurrent FSGS patients, the study showed elevated factor levels in recurrent post-transplant FSGS. Recurrent FSGS patient serum significantly damaged podocytes, reducing intact stress fibers by up to 59%. Notably, new blocking antibodies anti-uPAR (2G10) and anti-CD40 (BMS-986090) prevented this damage [44]. These findings deepen our understanding of FSGS pathogenesis, suggesting new therapeutic strategies targeting suPAR and anti-CD40 antibodies, offering hope for more effective future treatments [44].

4.4 Cytokines

Cardiotrophin-like cytokine factor-1 (CLCF-1): CLCF-1, a pleiotropic cytokine in the IL-6 family, is produced by various cells and tissues, including monocytes, macrophages, activated T cells, lymph nodes, spleen, bone marrow, peripheral blood lymphocytes, ovary, placenta, kidney, pituitary, and fetal liver [71]. CLCF-1, with a 22 kDa molecular weight, promotes B-cell expansion and antibody production, potentially including podocyte-targeting antibodies. CLCF-1 is a potential circulating permeability factor in primary FSGS [45, 72]. Its podocyte damage mechanism involves CLCF-1 interacting with apical domains of podocyte pedicels extending through GBM pores in direct plasma contact, binding to apical CNTFRα/gp130/LIFRβ complex, activating JAK2, phosphorylating and activating STAT3 translocating to the nucleus, and regulating various gene transcription. Some genes may encode proteins involved in actin cytoskeleton organization, like nephrin, podocin, or synaptopodin. JAK2 may directly phosphorylate key podocyte cytoskeleton proteins like actin, α-actinin-4, or synaptopodin, altering their assembly, stability, or interactions, disrupting normal cytoskeleton architecture. JAK2 activation may cross-activate other signaling pathways regulating the cytoskeleton, like PI3K/Akt, MAPK, or Rho GTPases pathways, controlling actin dynamics, cellular contractility, and motility [45, 46]. Proposed therapeutic approaches include JAK2 or STAT3 inhibitors and oral galactose therapy, with contradictory results [47, 73].

Soluble urokinase plasminogen activator receptor (suPAR): suPAR, a soluble form of urokinase receptor, originates from activated immune cells, including neutrophils, monocytes, and lymphocytes [74]. With a 55–60 kDa molecular weight, suPAR is implicated in FSGS pathogenesis by activating αvβ3 integrin signaling in podocytes, resulting in podocyte foot process effacement and proteinuria [48, 75]. However, suPAR's role as a specific FSGS biomarker remains controversial, with contradictory study results [49, 50]. No specific suPAR-based FSGS treatment has been established. Other studies questioned suPAR's specificity as an rFSGS biomarker, with elevated levels observed in other conditions, including general renal dysfunction. Despite promising initial results, suPAR's diagnostic and prognostic utility in FSGS is questioned due to lack of specificity and variability among studies. suPAR levels may be influenced by renal function, complicating interpretation in advanced renal disease patients [66].

Hemopexin: Hemopexin (Hpx) is a 60 kDa plasma glycoprotein primarily produced by the liver, though glomerular mesangial cells can synthesize it in response to inflammatory stimuli like TNF-α [51, 52]. Several studies suggest Hpx might act as a "circulating permeability factor" in FSGS. Purified Hpx has serum protease activity affecting glomerular podocyte structure and function. In vitro studies showed Hpx induces nephrin-dependent actin cytoskeleton reorganization in podocytes, leading to foot process loss and increased glomerular permeability. In animal models, purified Hpx infusion induced reversible proteinuria and FSGS-like glomerular changes in rats [52]. In post-transplant recurrent FSGS context, some studies detected elevated Hpx plasma levels in recurrence patients. Plasma Hpx activity is proposed as a potential biomarker for recurrence prediction. Ex vivo experiments showed rFSGS patient plasma induces Hpx-mediated podocyte damage in cell cultures. A reported case showed FSGS patient's kidney transplant to another non-FSGS recipient resolved proteinuria, suggesting a circulating factor like Hpx [53]. Proposed Hpx action mechanisms in FSGS include direct podocyte damage, JNK/SAPK and NFκB signaling pathway activation, oxidative stress induction, and glomerular filtration barrier alteration. Interestingly, pre-incubation with normal human plasma inhibited Hpx's harmful effect on podocytes in vitro, suggesting protective factors in normal plasma potentially diminished in FSGS [54]. Hpx activity modulation as a therapeutic approach in FSGS is actively researched. Approaches include serum protease inhibitors, anti-Hpx antibodies, and plasma protective factor mimetics. However, Hpx's exact role in FSGS remains controversial. Some studies found no significant Hpx level differences between FSGS patients and controls [76]. Recent proteomic studies identified Hpx as a potential urinary biomarker differentiating between mild and progressive FSGS forms. Severe FSGS patients showed elevated urinary Hpx levels with other podocyte damage and complement activation markers, reinforcing Hpx's potential role in FSGS pathogenesis and progression [77].

Interleukin-13 (IL-13): IL-13 is a 12–13 kDa cytokine produced by Th2, CD4+, and CD8+ T cells [55, 56, 78]. IL-13 has emerged as a potentially important factor in pFSGS and rFSGS pathogenesis. Various studies have provided significant evidence of IL-13's role in this renal disease. Studies demonstrated increased IL-13 expression in FSGS patients. Yap et al. found higher IL-13 mRNA expression in CD4+ and CD8+ T cells from relapsing SSNS children compared to remission [55]. These findings suggest IL-13 might be involved in disease pathogenesis, potentially acting as a circulating factor affecting podocyte function. IL-13 appears to have direct effects on glomerular podocytes. Van den Berg et al. demonstrated IL-13 receptor expression on human and rat podocytes [57]. IL-13-stimulated cultured podocytes showed decreased transepithelial electrical resistance, suggesting increased permeability. These in vitro findings provide a potential mechanism for IL-13's contribution to FSGS-characteristic glomerular filtration barrier dysfunction. A significant advance in understanding IL-13's role in FSGS came from developing an IL-13 overexpression rat model by Lai et al. [57]. IL-13 transfected rats developed FSGS-like characteristics, including proteinuria, hypoalbuminemia, hyperlipidemia, and foot process effacement resembling minimal change nephropathy. Molecularly, decreased glomerular nephrin, podocin, and dystroglycan expression was observed, proteins key to maintaining the glomerular filtration barrier. Increased glomerular B7-1 (CD80) expression in response to IL-13 was also observed, potentially contributing to slit diaphragm destabilization. Although evidence is more limited in post-transplant FSGS, IL-13 is suggested to be involved in post-transplant disease recurrence. Elevated serum IL-13 levels could act as a circulating factor affecting podocyte function in the transplanted kidney, though further studies are needed to confirm this hypothesis and establish clinical relevance. Identifying IL-13 as a pathogenic factor in FSGS opens new therapeutic possibilities. Blocking IL-13 or its signaling pathways could be a promising strategy for treating primary and recurrent FSGS. However, clinical studies are needed to validate this approach and determine efficacy and safety in patients.

Tumor necrosis factor-alpha (TNF-α): TNF-α is a pleiotropic cytokine produced by various cells, including macrophages, T cells, natural killer (NK) cells, neutrophils, mast cells, eosinophils, and neurons. It exists in two forms: a 17 kDa soluble form and a 26 kDa transmembrane form [79]. TNF-α induces podocyte injury through TNF signaling pathway activation in podocytes, leading to TNF-α expression upregulation in podocytes, perpetuating damage [58, 80]. Precise mechanisms of TNF-α altering podocyte function are not fully characterized. Anti-TNF-α monoclonal antibodies like adalimumab have shown some efficacy in reducing proteinuria in an FSGS patient subgroup [59]. TNF pathway activation in cultured podocytes exposed to FSGS patient sera may serve as a biomarker identifying patients who may benefit from anti-TNF-α therapy [58].

B cell activating factor (BAFF): BAFF, also known as BLyS or TNFSF13B, is a TNF family cytokine produced by monocytes, activated neutrophils, T cells, and dendritic cells [81, 82]. With a 31–35 kDa molecular weight, BAFF plays a crucial role in B-cell selection, survival, and maturation [60]. BAFF overexpression leads to autoreactive B-cell clone survival, resulting in autoantibody production [61, 81]. In FSGS, BAFF may contribute to pathogenesis by promoting autoreactive B cell survival and maturation, leading to autoantibody production against podocyte antigens [62]. BAFF also interacts with the complement system and T cells to amplify the immune response and podocyte injury [63, 83]. Belimumab, a monoclonal antibody targeting BAFF, has shown efficacy in reducing proteinuria in other autoantibody-mediated glomerular diseases like lupus nephritis [84, 85]. However, its efficacy in primary FSGS has not been established.

These permeability factors, including anti-nephrin, anti-UCH-L1, and anti-CD40 antibodies, sCD40L, CLCF-1, suPAR, Hpx, IL-13, TNF-α, BAFF, and others, are implicated in primary and post-transplant recurrent FSGS pathogenesis. Further studies in well-characterized patient cohorts and in vivo animal models are needed to fully elucidate precise mechanisms and develop targeted therapies for each permeability factor or their removal through therapeutic plasma exchange (TPE) or immunoadsorption [85].

5. Clinical and histological course

The term true recurrence should be reserved for native kidney biopsies and post-renal transplant biopsies, which makes their evaluation difficult due to their availability [86].

rFSGS is a pathological term used to indicate glomerular lesion associated with various etiological factors (2), recurrence of FSGS in renal allografts is a major cause of graft loss [87].

The clinical characteristics of rFSGS are quite heterogeneous, English et al. show us the most salient symptoms reported were tiredness, swelling, shortness of breath, loss of appetite, and dry, itchy skin.

"Fatigue" was the most common response to symptoms, reported by the majority of patients, with a profound negative impact on activities of daily living being one of the most worrying symptoms [88]. But there is a common denominator, which is proteinuria, hematuria, and deterioration of renal function. The intensity of each clinical characteristic depends on the etiology, the time of appearance of post-transplant proteinuria, and its association with graft rejection, immunosuppression or de novo glomerulonephritis.

Classically, it is understood that clinical manifestations could be characterized according to the time of early onset within 48–72 hours after the transplant typically with massive proteinuria and late onset with a phenotype of progressive nephrotic syndrome developed in the months or years after surgery [86]. The frequent occurrence of proteinuria within a few hours or days after transplantation suggests that podocyte injury is probably caused by a factor of circulating permeability [25], when severe proteinuria occurred within 3 months after transplantation, Taneda et al. showed the collapsing variant, while the not otherwise specified variant became more common 2 years after transplant [89].

In children, the median time for recurrent proteinuria is approximately 10 to 14 days after transplantation while in adults, and the median time for recurrence is approximately 1.5 months [16, 90–92].

Therefore, the interval between the transplant and the onset of rFSGS symptoms can change, but it is estimated that if it occurs during the first year, the condition is more severe. Accurate evaluation of FSGS lesions is required to facilitate diagnosis and clinical management [89]. According to Taneda et al., the collapsing variant may occur by podocyte injury and also by endothelial injury or disruption of epithelium and endothelium crosstalk, which may relate to the molecular mechanisms involved, treatment, and prognosis. There is no evidence to suggest that minimal levels of immunosuppression correlate with histological findings, but among the multiple causes of FSGS, the secondary was the most common FSGS in grafts [87].

6. Pretransplant risk prediction

It is important to know the risk factors and their mechanism of action since they can and have an impact on graft survival; its objective is to develop effective strategies for its prevention and management.

Several risk factors associated with the recurrence of FSGS have been described, most of them are non-modifiable factors; their prevalence and distribution varies according to the type of population according to the literature as described in the

Risk factor of recurrence	Grade	p-value	Reference
Younger age of the recipients	IR	(p = 0.001)	[15, 93]
Rapid progression to ESRD	IR	(p = 0.018)	[15, 94]
Mesangial proliferation in the native kidney biopsy (reflecting a more severe form of disease) and steroid resistance	IR		[95]
Older donor; protective factor (p = 0,008) (11)	IR		[96]
Pre-transplant bilateral nephrectomy	No data	(OR 6.53, IC 95% 2.68–15.92, p < 0.001)	[15, 22]
Recurrence of FSGS in a previous allograft	IR		[97]
White than in non-Caucasian patients	IR		[17]
Idiopathic FSGS	No data		[98]
Living-related donation compared with deceased donor, particularly in the pediatric recipients	IR	(p 0.007)	[15, 17]
Increased levels of soluble urokinase-type plasminogen activator receptor (suPAR)	No data		[48]
Antibodies that may be related with recurrent FSGS: CD40 (correlated with a greater risk of recurrence), PTPRO, CGB5, FAS, P2RY11, SNRPB2, and APOL2	LR		[70]
Familial FSGS, no significant association was found between HLA.	LR	(OR – 0.17, IC 95% -0.37 - 0.04, p = 0.107)	[15, 99]
Sporadic form with podocin mutation	LR		[99]
Slow progressive to uremia	LR		[99]
Non-nephrotic proteinuria in the original disease.	LR		[99]
A higher level of proteinuria before transplantation has been associated with a higher risk of FSGS recurrence	IR	(p < .001)	[99]

Low risk = LR.
Increased risk = IR.

Table 4.
Risk factor of recurrence.

following table. It should be noted that we also found protective factors, although there is a high level of evidence to prove the contrary, according to the literature reviewed, see **Table 4**.

7. Prophylactic therapy to prevent recurrence of FSGS prior to transplantation

Recurrence has been associated with early graft loss, which is why different prophylactic therapy schemes have been proposed. Unfortunately, multinational randomized controlled studies with a homogeneous treatment protocol are still required (**Table 5**).

Recently, a systematic review was carried out to assess the benefit of rituximab, with or without plasmapheresis, compared to standard treatment. A total of 11 studies (399 patients) were analyzed. There was no significant difference in recurrence

Author	Study	n	Type of prophylactic	Results
Kwon et al. [100]	Single-center retrospective	99	No TPE vs. TPE	No pre-treatment group (16 [34.8%]) FSGS recurrence vs. pre-treatment group (5 [9.4%]; P = 0.002)
Mariarosaria Campise et al. [101]	Single-center retrospective study	42	21 received prophylactic TPE 10 received posttransplant prophylactic TPE 11 received pre- and posttransplant prophylactic TPE	Comparison between this series and a historical control group of 52 patients with primary focal segmental glomerulosclerosis transplanted and not receiving plasmapheresis prophylaxis did not demonstrate any advantages
Sami Alasfar et al. [92]	Prospective observational study	66	TPE and/or rituximab	62% who received preventative therapy developed recurrence compared to 51% who did not receive any therapy (p = 0.21)
Gohh et al. [102]	Prospective observational study	19	TPE	Recurrence rates of 60% were expected if no treatment was given
Ohta, Toshiyuki et al. [103]	Retrospective study	21	15 prophylactic PP vs. 6 no prophylactic TPE	TPE appears to be effective for the prevention and treatment of posttransplant recurrence of FSGS
Boonpheng B et al. [104]	Systematic review and meta-analysis	399	399 rituximab studies), 571 (plasmapheresis studies) rituximab with or without plasmapheresis, and plasmapheresis alone.	No significant difference in FSGS recurrence between rituximab (with or without plasmapheresis) and standard treatment (RR 0.82, 95% CI: 0.47–1.45). No significant difference between plasmapheresis alone and no plasmapheresis (RR 0.85, 95% CI: 0.60–1.21).

Table 5.
Prophylactic therapy to prevent recurrence of FSGS.

with a pooled risk of 0.82 (95%CI: 0.47–1.45, I^2 = 65%), and similarly, no significant difference was evident in the group with only plasmapheresis versus no plasmapheresis 0.85 (95%CI: 0.60–1.21, I^2 = 23%).

Subgroup analysis in the pediatric and adult groups did not reveal a significant difference in the risk of recurrence. Significant changes post-transplant were observed, including timing of recurrence and graft survival [104].

The potential for positive publication bias and the absence of RCT (randomized controlled trial) evidence make prognostic information speculative. Therefore, the optimal therapeutic approach is not well known and treatment strategies vary among transplant centers.

8. Treatment of recurrent FSGS

Primary focal segmental glomerulosclerosis (FSGS) recurs in up to 55% of patients after kidney transplantation, which could be divided depending on the time of recurrency, into early (less than 3 months), which is characterized by massive proteinuria days after transplantations or weeks before it, or late recurrency (more than 3 months). It is demonstrated that it significantly increases allograft loss, leading to morbidity and mortality. Management of both forms still represents a challenge nowadays, and there are no consensus guidelines for the management of recurrent FSGS; therefore, the treatment remains largely empirical.

There must be recognized, high risk factors for recurrence, some of them listed as younger age, rapid progression of the disease to end-stage renal disease on native kidneys, and loss of previous renal allografts due to recurrence.

Most of transplantation groups prefer using the term multitarget therapy in recurrent disease, as it shows the bibliography below.

8.1 Corticosteroid

Corticosteroids constitute the first line treatment of primary focal segmental glomerular esclerosis, its effects target multiple sites involving mainly nephrin and podocine proteins.

As mentioned above, nephrin is the key component of the slit diaphragm which is a protein with an extracellular and intracellular domain, its main function serves as a filter and preserves the normal structure of the podocyte. It is also anchored to the membrane cell and to the cytoskeleton by the podocine protein and by the CD2-associated protein (CD2AP), respectively. When it is about podocyte injury, in rat models, it is been demonstrated that the injury pathway involves decreased phosphorylation, which is restored after glucocorticoid treatment, consisting its primary effect in phosphorylation of nephrin. These effect increases prosurvival signaling via CD2AP and α-tubulin; inducing olfactomedin domain protein 1 (Olfm 1) that stabilizes the actin cytoskeleton [105]. Nephrin phosphorylation is achieved by activating serum and glucocorticoid-regulated kinase 1 (SGK1) and Src family kinases.

Another profound effect in the regulation of podocine and nephrine is by the transcription factor (nuclear) krüppel-like factor 15 (KLF 15), which is been directly related with corticoid responsiveness [106]. This factor decreases nuclear factor of activated T cell (NFAT) signaling, enhancing the expression of specific genes such as NEPHS1 and NEPHS2, and controls retinoic acid which is essential in differentiation of other molecules as podocine and synaptopodine, directly related to FSGS proteinuria.

Other proteins like caveolin-1 (CAV-1) and transient receptor potential channel 6 (TRPC6) act as a mechanical stress, and corticosteroids induce downregulation of this protein diminishing mechanical pressure changes in podocyte, binding directly this receptor, and blocking its signal pathway, leading to stabilization of the slit diafragm [107].

Downregulation of CD80 protein is also well known to be an effect of corticosteroids therapy, blocking its effect mediated through the activation of toll-like receptor 3 (TLR 3), which is involved in the induction of proinflammatory response [108].

RhoA protein is positively expressed with glucorticoids, and its presence is crucial for synaptopodine stability. In contrast, Ras-related C3 botulinum toxin substrate 1 (RAC 1) is an important regulator of synaptodine, and its presence is related to the instability of synaptopodine. Corticosteroids downregulate RAC 1 expression and cGMP which are both enhanced by each other [109].

Referring to cytoskeleton organization, there are other proteins like focal adhesion kinase (FAK) which binds to actin and B1 integrin, and its action through RANKL protein activates downstream mediators that lead to apoptosis of the podocyte cell [110].

Actinin-α-4 is an actin crosslinking protein, another key protein that stabilizes the podocyte cytoskeleton. It has been experimentally demonstrated that its expression is augmented in patients with nephrotic syndrome [111], activating pro-apoptotic pathways and overexpression of angptl4 which is inhibited as well by corticosteroid therapy [111]. These drugs simultaneously induce recruitment and attachment of actinin-α-4 to certain transactivated gene bindings sites in the nucleus, like serpin family E member 1 (SERPINE 1), angiopoietin-like 4 (ANGPTL4), chemokine (C-C motif) ligand 20 (CCL20), and serum amyloid A1 (SAA1) [112, 113]. Since these genes are linked to certain pathways that encode, like SERPINE 1, glucocorticoids indirectly activate some adverse effects, as plasminogen activator inhibitor 1(PAI 1), which is known to be responsible for some of the adverse effects of this drugs, related to albuminuria and glomerulosclerosis [114]. Another molecule which also mediates proteinuria is CCL20. All these genes are related with inflammation in diabetic kidney disease.

Corticosteroid therapy alter small group of non-coding RNAs that regulate post-transcriptional gene expression (microRNA), and its expression which is upregulated by the therapy reduces apoptotic signaling pathways (diminishes cellular tumor antigen p53) [115]. Its effects in downregulating proinflammatory pathways is well-known such as inducing downstream of certain interleukins (IL6, IL 8, IL 11, and IL23A), chemokines (CCL 2 and CXCL 12), TFG-ß1, Interferon regulatory factors (IRF 2 IRF6), tumor necrosis factor, and colony stimulating factor (CSF2) [116].

Its crucial role in multiple targets in podocyte makes corticosteroids a cornerstone therapy that cannot be excluded.

8.2 Antiproliferative agents

Mycophenolate mofetil is a prodrug of mycophenolate acid (MPA), which is a reversible uncompetitive inhibitor of inositol monophospathe dehydrogenase (IMDH), an enzyme that plays a main role in synthesis of purine de novo with the consequent proliferation of T and B cells. Because of this inhibition, it plays a fundamental role suppressing T-cell-mediated response and antibody formation by activated B cells.

Its other effects non-immune-mediated have to do with avoiding the proliferation of mesangial cells, expansion of mesangial matrix and foot process effacement of podocytes. Since mesangial cells are partially dependent on the novo purine synthesis, they respond to MPA action [117].

MPA modifies pathway sequesters of ATP consumption, which is needed for RNA and DNA synthesis needed for the expression of actin and synaptopodyn proteins and maintaining cytoskeleton homeostasis [105].

In podocyte cells, MPA attenuates the expression of urokinase receptors (uPAR) mRNA protein levels, and these molecules lead to a downstream signal pathway responsible for foot process effacement via loss protein lipid-dependent activation of alfa beta 3 integrin; these effects were shown in lupus nephritis mice models though. Still needing studies in FSGS [48].

Reduce the apoptosis of podocytes through a reduction of Bax and cleaved caspase 3 protein levels (CC3). Reduce the activation of RAC 1 on cultured podocytes experimentally treated [118].

This effect of MPA is also seen in glucose-enriched murine podocytes, regulating the expression of cell cycle protein p27(kip1), p21(cip1), avoiding the hypertrophy of podocytes, which is a consequence of the upregulation of p27 and p21 under diabetic conditions; however, these effects were not been demonstrated in FSGS [119]. These proteins, besides, upstream angiotensin II, known to cause hypertrophy of mesangial and tubular cells. And, in podocytes, angiotensin II mediates rearrangement of the actin cytoskeleton, depolarization, and increase in cytosolic calcium activity and apoptosis.

Also, it has been demonstrated that MPA causes downregulation of many inflammatory pathways, like p38-mitogen-activated protein kinase (p38MAPK) and nuclear factor kappa-beta (Nf-kb).

MMF treatment diminishes early renal injury via the inhibition of oxidative stress and overexpression of ICAM-1, MCP-1, and TGF-beta1 in renal tissue in diabetic rats, molecules related to adhesion of macrophages and monocytes, and propagation of inflammation, key pattern in stress changes on podocytes [119, 120]. Some of these molecules implicated with oxidative stress like malondialdehyde (MDA) and TGF-beta1 were demonstrated to be annulled in experimental studies by MPA. In other studies, MMF inhibits the upregulation of CD18 in lymphocytes, contributing as well to the infiltration of monocytes.

A multicenter, randomized, controlled trial assessed whether treatment with mycophenolate mofetil (MMF) and oral pulses of dexamethasone (DEXA) was more effective treatment than cyclosporine alone for steroid-resistant FSGS. They concluded that the incidence of complete and partial remissions was 33% in the MMF and DEXA group compared with 46% in the cyclosporine group (inferior), [121]. Another study 6 months open label where it was used MMF in 18 patients with biopsy proven steroid-resistant FSGS, proteinuria diminished in 44% [122].

8.3 Calcineurin inhibitors

Calcineurin (CN) is a calcium and calmodulin-dependent serine/threonine phosphatase that activates the nuclear factor of activated T cells (NFAT), by dephosphorylating it. Then, this molecule is translocated to the nucleus leading to transcriptional activation of cytokine genes and also activating T-cell-induced immune response. The CN inhibitors (CNIs) like tacrolimus and cyclosporine A (CsA) are immunosuppressive drugs used in organ transplantation widely and in glomerulonephritis also. These agents decrease production of cytokines such as IL-2 and IL-4, by inhibiting the activation of NFAT in T cells.

Angiopoietin-like-4 (ANGPTL4) is a well-known protein that is implicated in the generation of proteinuria in podocyte-related nephropathy. Shen et al. cultured podocytes of rat models with proteinuria induced by puromycin aminonucleoside (PAN)-induced minimal-change disease (MCD). In this study, they demonstrated that CaN inhibitors protected against PAN-induced podocyte injury, by inhibition of Nfatc1 and Angptl4 in vivo and in vitro [123]. Angptl4 directly induced rearrangement of the cytoskeleton of the podocytes, reducing the expression of synaptopodin, and enhanced PAN-induced podocyte apoptosis, increasing the pro-apoptotic proteins Bax and cleaved caspase-3. Also, this molecule is related to adipose metabolism, inhibiting liporprotein lipase activity which leads to hypertriglyceridemia; wound repair, and tumor metastasis; and is controlled by factors like TGF-β, PPAR, and HIF-1α which are segregated mainly in peripheral tissues. It has been seen that genetic polymorphisms of ANGPTL4 have been associated with the severity of post-transplant proteinuria in kidney allograft recipients.

Specifically, it has been shown that cyclosporin A prevents synaptopodin from cathepsin-L-mediated degradation, and cytosolic CatL proteolyzes synaptopodin and results in disorganization of podocyte actin cytoskeleton. Since this effect is blocked, it leads to the preservation of phosphorylated synaptopodin and subsequent RhoA-mediated stabilization of actin stress fibers under cell stress [124].

Another report revealed that CNI stabilized podocyte cytoskeleton by upregulating expression of cofilin, which was independent of its effect on synaptopodin [125]. Cofilins are essential proteins liable for the turnover and reorganization of actin filaments.

As described by Schlöndorff J et al., in aggressive forms of FSGS, there exists upregulation of TRPC6 channels because of mutations, which is related to augmented calcium influx in the podocyte cells activating the calcineurin pathway. Calcineurin inhibitors may also mitigate podocyte injury by reducing the intracellular influx of calcium. TRPC6 mutants are blocked by inhibitors of calcineurin, calmodulin-dependent kinase II, and phosphatidylinositol 3-kinase [126].

Also, was investigated the effect of tacrolimus on proteinuria in anti-nephrin antibody-induced nephropathy. Experimentally, Wakamatsu et al. demonstrated that this drug significantly ameliorate proteinuria in rats injected with anti-nephrin antibodies [127].

8.4 mTOR inhibitors

The immunosuppressive mammalian target of rapamycin (mTOR) inhibitors can cause proteinuria, especially in patients with kidney and heart transplant. Its main function role as a drug with growth-inhibitor capability and anti-tumor properties is well known [128].

Progression of focal segmental glomerulosclerosis (FSGS) is associated with podocyte loss and hypertrophy of remaining podocytes. "Complete mTOR inhibition or mTOR hyperactivation accelerates glomerulosclerosis progression, whereas moderate mTOR inhibition has a beneficial effect." According to Huber et al. [129]. The researchers noted the upregulation of mTORC1 target genes in microdissected glomeruli from patients with primary FSGS compared with levels in patients with minimal change disease. Similarly, mTORC1 was activated in podocytes of mice with adriamycin (ADR)-induced nephropathy, and this hyperactivation of mTORC1 led to the development of FSGS-like lesions, highlighting this receptor mTORC1 activation as a driver of FSGS.

Recent researches, have shown that podocyte size control is regulated by mammalian target of rapamycin (mTOR) [130], and mTOR activation contribute to progression of glomerular disease. There is a serine/threonine kinase of the mTOR, which catalyzes this drug into two subunits, mTOR complex 1 and 2 (mTORC1 and mTORC2). The activation of mTORC1 results into direct phosphorylation of the ribosomal S6 kinase (S6K) and the eukaryotic translation initiation factor 4E–binding protein (4E-BP), which stimulates ribosome biogenesis and protein translation to increase cell mass [131]. So, the principal target of mTOR inhibitor is mTORC1, in steroid-resistant FSGS and FSGS recurrence after kidney transplantation, and it has been reported both successful and deleterious, indicating an incomplete understanding of the role of the mTOR pathway in this glomerular disease [132].

Sirolimus is a structural analogue of tacrolimus, as it binds to the same immunophilin FKPB12 receptors but does not alter calcineurin phosphatase activity. When the drug reaches target levels, it blocks cytokine-dependent T-cell proliferation at the G1-S phase of the cell cycle. Some authors used this drug for treatment of glomerulonephritis, one of them, Fervenza et al. [30], who used sirolimus in six patients with various forms of chronic glomerulonephritis, and he found increased serum creatinine after 12 months of therapy. Another work of Tumlim et al. [133] found that sirolimus stabilized renal function in patients with FSGS, on contrary to Fervenza, after 12 months of therapy, demonstrating increase in serum creatinine by <10% among the sirolimus-responsive patients compared with a doubling of serum creatinine between resistant patients. Likewise in another experimental study, Zschiedrich et al. [131] showed that murine glomerular disease models with FSGS showed that the complete knockout of mTORC1 by induced deletion of both Raptor alleles accelerated the progression of murine FSGS models. However, lowering mTORC1 signaling by deleting just one Raptor allele ameliorated the progression of glomerulosclerosis. Concluding that low-dose treatment with the mTORC1 inhibitor, rapamycin efficiently diminished disease progression.

8.5 Cyclophosphamide

Cyclophosphamide has been reported to be associated with varying response rates in the treatment of rFSGS. Used as induction therapy, Kershaw et al. reported a complete remission in two of three patients and partial remission in one of three patients [134]. Two studies used cyclophosphamide as a substitute for an antimetabolite medication post-transplant concurrently with TPE and pulse corticosteroids, and this led to sustained rFSGS remission in all three patients in one study but only 33% of 16 children in the other study [134, 135]. In another report, cyclophosphamide and TPE alone produced a sustained remission in seven of 11 patients [136].

8.6 Rituximab

Rituximab (RTX) is a chimeric monoclonal IgG1 antibody that targets the CD20 receptor expressed on B lymphocytes and depletes B cells through the Fcγ immunoglobulin receptor (FcγR), complement, and apoptotic pathways. Its main use is for hematologic malignancies, but recently, its use in glomerulopathies is widespread specially when it comes to the podocytes [105].

Rituximab treatment of high-risk FSGS patients has been associated with lower incidence of post-transplant proteinuria and might prevent recurrent FSGS after kidney transplantation, potentially through a direct regulation of podocyte function, as rituximab directly preserves sphingomyelin phosphodiesterase acid-like 3b (SMPDL-3b) and ASMase activity in podocytes. Even though CD20 mRNA nor protein which are expressed in B cells (target of Rtx) are not present in podocytes. RTx binds to podocyte cells trough SMPDL-3b regulating likewise acid-sphingomyelinase (ASMase) activity, which regulates the conversion of sphingomyelin to ceramide [137].

In a French retrospective multicenter study, Lanaret et al. [138] showed that, from 148 transplant recipients with FSGS diagnosis, in which RTX was used along with plasmapheresis, it could be used in cases where standard of care therapy with plasmapheresis, plus high doses of cyclosporine A, plus high doses of corticosteroids; failed or for early discontinuation of plasmapheresis, without increasing the risk of infections. This French cohort of FSGS treatment was largely inspired by the strategy of multitarget therapy described by Canaud et al. consisting in high doses of oral steroids during 4 weeks with subsequent tapering, intravenous cyclosporine during 2 weeks, followed by oral treatment and plasmapheresis with 5% albumin reposition three sessions per week during 3 weeks followed by two sessions per week for 3 weeks, then one session per week until month 3, then two sessions per month until month 5, and finally one a month until month 9 [139].

In another meta-analysis, Boonpheng et al. [104] assessed that the risk of recurrence of FSGS using prophylactic rituximab with or without plasmapheresis, or plasmapheresis alone, where the use of rituximab with or without plasmapheresis, or plasmapheresis alone, is not associated with a lower risk of FSGS recurrence after kidney transplantation. Future studies are required to assess the effectiveness of rituximab with or without plasmapheresis among specific patient subgroups with high-risk for FSGS recurrence. In a subgroup analysis, four studies with patients deemed to be at high-risk of recurrence, based on demographic and clinical criteria, and only Fornoni et al. [137] showed a significantly lower recurrence risk in the rituximab group. On the contrary, the remaining three studies with the same patients reported a numerically higher recurrence in the rituximab group [92, 140, 141].

Another recent meta-analysis evaluated the efficacy of combined rituximab and plasmapheresis (or plasma exchange) in patients with recurrent FSGS after kidney transplantation. The combination therapy of rituximab and plasmapheresis resulted in an overall remission rate of 72.7% (95% CI 52.3–86.6%). Complete remission was 41.0% of patients, while 31.7% achieved partial remission. The treatment led to a significant reduction in proteinuria and serum creatinine levels. This combined approach appears promising for managing recurrent FSGS, but individual patient responses may vary [142].

8.7 Sodium-glucose cotransporter-2 inhibitors

Within the pharmacodynamics and pharmacokinetics of sodium-glucose cotransporter-2 inhibitors (SGLT2i), there are two glucose transporters that are important for glucose reabsorption. Both are in the proximal tubules of the kidneys: sodium-glucose cotransporter 1 (SGLT1), located in the S3 segment of the proximal tubule; and sodium-glucose cotransporter 2 (SGLT2), located in the S1 segment of the proximal renal tubule. SGLT2 are responsible for the reabsorption of approximately 90% of filtered glucose [143].

The 2024 Kidney Disease: Improving Global Outcomes (KDIGO) guidelines for chronic kidney disease (June 2024) provide recommendations for the use of SGLT2i regardless of whether or not the patient has diabetes [144].

The subanalysis of the DAPA-CKD study, with 104 participants with FSGS confirmed by kidney biopsy, demonstrated the advantage of SGLT2i, after modifying the estimated GFR (40% decrease) in the original DAPA-CKD study [145], when added to ACEi/ARB therapy, dapagliflozin reduced the rate of chronic eGFR decline over a median of 2.4 years treatment [146]. In the Empagliflozin Heart and Kidney Protection Study (EMPA-KIDNEY), the benefit of empagliflozin was greatest in patients with an albumin/creatinine ratio ≥ 300 mg/g and substantially less in patients with lower albumin excretion [147].

Among the general measures for the treatment of recurrent FSGS and SGLT2i are described, it is already known for their renal protective benefits in patients with proteinuric chronic kidney disease (with or without diabetes). They can also be beneficial in transplant recipients with recurrent FSGS, although studies with greater statistical power are lacking [148, 149].

Boeckhaus et al. report data in a series of cases of patients with Alport syndrome and focal segmental glomerulosclerosis (FSGS) with respect to the early effect of SGLT2i on kidney function. Mean urinary albumin-creatinine ratio in mg/g creatinine before SGLT2i initiation was 1827 (1560) and decreased by almost 40% to 1127 (854) after SGLT2i initiation [150].

It is important to mention the association of SGLT2i in patients who maintain immunosuppressive therapies. There are cases reported in patients with glomerular diseases maintained immunosuppressive therapies to evaluate the safety of their use. Elkeraie et al., in an open and uncontrolled study, during a mean period of 7.3 months of follow-up, mentions that the incidence rate of urinary tract infection (UTI) was 1.6 per 100 person-months. UTI episodes were successfully treated with antibiotic therapy without the need to discontinue SGLT2i. There were no cases of acute kidney injury (AKI), ketoacidosis, amputation, nor Fournier's gangrene. It concludes that SGLT2i is safe to use in patients with glomerular diseases on immunosuppressive therapies, but there are no studies in kidney transplant recipients [151].

8.8 ACE inhibitors and ARBs

Increased expression of nuclear factor-kB and the angiotensinogen gene has been observed in patients with rFSGS [152]. In mouse models, where it was hypothesized that angiotensin II may contribute to rFSGS by causing preferential constriction of the afferent arteriole and associated increased intraglomerular pressure [153].

Many case series have reported the antiproteinuric efficacy of renin-angiotensin system blockers in rFSGS [154, 155]. Abuzeineh et al. found an association of angiotensin II type 1 receptors and rFSGS, leading to worse allograft outcome.

It is the recommended therapy with angiotensin-converting enzyme inhibitors or angiotensin receptor blockers in patients with persistent proteinuria in the absence of contraindications, with close monitoring of kidney function (2C) [6].

9. New treatments

9.1 Ofatumumab

Ofatumumab is a second-generation, fully human anti-CD20 monoclonal antibody. Unlike rituximab, which is a chimeric (murine/human) antibody, ofatumumab is entirely human [156, 157].

The mechanism of action of ofatumumab involves binding to the CD20 antigen on the surface of B lymphocytes. It has a higher affinity for the CD20 epitope compared to rituximab and causes a more prolonged depletion of B cells. It induces greater complement-dependent cytotoxicity and dissociates more slowly from the CD20 receptor. Additionally, it more potently activates antibody-dependent cell-mediated cytotoxicity (ADCC) and antibody-dependent cellular phagocytosis (ADCP) [156–158].

Results in patients with recurrent post-transplant FSGS have been variable. It has been used primarily in pediatric cases resistant to rituximab and plasmapheresis. In a series of six pediatric patients, none achieved complete remission, 3/6 (50%) achieved partial remission, and 3/6 (50%) did not respond [158]. In an individual pediatric case, sustained partial remission was achieved for 13 months [159]. In a series of seven patients (five pediatric, two adult), 4/5 pediatric patients achieved partial or complete response, but neither of the two adult patients responded [160].

The use of ofatumumab in adults with recurrent post-transplant FSGS is limited, with few cases reported in the literature. In one case of a 44-year-old adult with recurrent FSGS resistant to plasmapheresis, rituximab, and abatacept, late partial remission (at 9 months) was achieved and maintained for 30 months of follow-up after ofatumumab administration. This patient received a total dose of 700 mg (500 mg/m2) in four doses at 2-week intervals, which is a lower dose than that used in pediatric studies [161].

The response appears to be better in the pediatric population than in adults. In some cases, the response can be delayed, up to 9 months after treatment. The doses used have been variable, ranging from 500 to 1500 to 2000 mg/m^2. Reported adverse effects have generally been mild, mainly minor allergic reactions [158–161].

9.2 Abatacept and belatacept

Abatacept is a fusion protein composed of the Fc region of IgG1 fused to the extracellular domain of CTLA-4. It acts as a selective costimulation modulator by binding to CD80 and CD86 on antigen-presenting cells, thereby inhibiting the CD28-mediated costimulation of T cells. Abatacept was initially reported to induce remission in five patients with recurrent FSGS after 1–2 doses. It was proposed to work by binding to B7-1 (CD80) expressed on podocytes in FSGS. However, subsequent studies have shown inconsistent results [162–164].

In one study of nine patients, abatacept failed to induce remission in any patients. Another study of 6 pediatric patients showed partial remission in 3/6 patients. A case report showed partial remission after 4 doses given over 4–6 weeks. Overall, results have been mixed and less promising than initially reported [162–165].

Belatacept is a second-generation CTLA-4 fusion protein with 2–4 fold higher binding affinity to CD80/CD86 compared to abatacept. Like abatacept, it inhibits T-cell costimulation by binding CD80/CD86. Belatacept has been proposed as a maintenance immunosuppression option to potentially prevent/treat recurrent FSGS, based on its higher binding affinity to B7-1 compared to abatacept [165, 166].

One case report showed successful long-term remission when belatacept was used as maintenance therapy after initial abatacept treatment. However, a case series of five patients showed no significant improvement in proteinuria with belatacept treatment. 2/5 patients in this series progressed to dialysis despite belatacept therapy [165, 166].

Both abatacept and belatacept have shown inconsistent results in treating recurrent FSGS after transplantation. While there are some case reports of success, larger case series have failed to show consistent benefit. The initial promising results with abatacept have not been widely reproduced. More research is needed to determine if there is a role for costimulation blockade in recurrent FSGS and to identify which patients may benefit from this approach. The mechanisms behind any potential benefit also require further elucidation, as B7-1 expression on podocytes has not been consistently demonstrated in FSGS [162–166].

9.3 Anti-tumor necrosis factor-alpha (TNFα)

Anti-TNF therapies work by blocking the effects of TNFα on podocytes. TNFα has been shown to disrupt the podocyte cytoskeleton, disperse focal adhesion complexes, and activate β3 integrin in podocytes. These effects likely contribute to podocyte detachment and proteinuria in FSGS. Anti-TNF agents can reverse these changes in vitro, restoring normal podocyte morphology and adhesion. TNFα binds to two receptors on podocytes – TNFRI (p55) and TNFRII (p75). Blocking either or both of these receptors with antibodies can prevent the toxic effects of FSGS plasma on cultured podocytes. TNFα signaling in podocytes leads to activation of NFκB, MAPK, Rho GTPases, and caspases, ultimately affecting the actin cytoskeleton and cell adhesion [167]. Anti-TNF therapies have shown promise in some cases of recurrent FSGS post-transplant that were resistant to other treatments. However, results have been inconsistent across studies. Leroy et al. reported the successful treatment of a case of biopsy-proven recurrent FSGS with infliximab at a dose of 3 mg/kg bimonthly along with high-dose corticosteroids (60 mg/1.73 m^2 per day). Notably, discontinuation of treatment led to relapses that were not controlled by corticosteroids or etanercept alone, suggesting a synergistic effect of combination therapy. Remission was achieved again when combination therapy was restarted. In another case report, a patient with recurrent FSGS resistant to plasmapheresis achieved partial remission with etanercept 0.5 mg/kg twice weekly, followed by infliximab 5 mg/kg monthly. This allowed discontinuation of plasmapheresis and led to sustained partial remission for over 11 months. Dosing regimens reported in the literature include etanercept 0.5 mg/kg twice weekly subcutaneously, infliximab 3–5 mg/kg intravenously every 4–8 weeks, and adalimumab 24 mg/m^2 every 2 weeks (maximum 40 mg) in primary FSGS. However, optimal dosing for recurrent FSGS has not been established. Treatment duration also varies, with some patients requiring long-term therapy to maintain remission. In vitro studies have shown that blocking TNFα or its receptors can reverse the effects of FSGS plasma on podocytes within 6 hours of treatment. This suggests that the beneficial effects may occur rapidly, but sustained therapy is likely needed to maintain remission in vivo. It is important to note that not all patients respond to anti-TNF therapy. In the FONT study of primary FSGS, only four out of 10 patients showed a response to adalimumab. The factors predicting response are not yet known. Anti-TNF therapies show promise for some cases of recurrent FSGS post-transplant, particularly those resistant to other treatments. However, more research is needed to determine optimal patient selection, dosing, and duration of therapy. The mechanisms of action on podocytes provide a rationale for their use, but clinical efficacy remains variable. Combination with other immunosuppressive agents may be necessary in some cases to achieve and maintain remission [167, 168].

9.4 Mesenchymal stromal cells

Mesenchymal stromal cells (MSCs) have demonstrated beneficial effects in podocyte and kidney repair in experimental models and some preliminary clinical studies of rFSGS after transplantation. The proposed mechanisms include paracrine effects, where MSCs secrete soluble factors and extracellular vesicles that promote podocyte survival and function. In one study, MSC treatment in mice with adriamycin-induced FSGS significantly reduced podocyte apoptosis and proteinuria, associated with a decrease in p-Smad3 expression in the glomeruli [169]. MSCs also have potent anti-inflammatory and immunomodulatory effects. In patients with recurrent post-transplant FSGS, MSC infusion was associated with a reduction in multiple circulating inflammatory factors, including CD40 ligand, IL-16, macrophage migration inhibitory factor, and myeloperoxidase [170]. Additionally, MSCs can inhibit renal fibrosis through the regulation of profibrotic pathways such as TGF-β/Smad. In the aforementioned study in mice with FSGS, MSC treatment significantly reduced the expression of p-Smad3, a key mediator of fibrosis [169]. Although not definitively demonstrated in FSGS, MSCs could activate endogenous renal progenitors to promote regeneration, as observed in other models of kidney injury. Regarding clinical results in recurrent post-transplant FSGS, a study of six pediatric patients with recurrent post-transplant FSGS resistant to conventional treatments, treatment with allogeneic MSCs resulted in partial remission in three patients (50%). Proteinuria was significantly reduced, and plasmapheresis could be discontinued in these patients [170].

A case report described a 13-year-old patient with recurrent post-transplant FSGS resistant to multiple therapies. After three infusions of allogeneic MSCs, sustained partial remission of proteinuria was achieved, allowing discontinuation of plasmapheresis. A significant reduction in multiple circulating inflammatory factors was observed, which was maintained for at least 1 year [170]. Another study reported the use of MSCs in two adult patients with recurrent post-transplant FSGS. One patient achieved complete remission and the other partial remission of proteinuria after MSC treatment [171]. These results, although preliminary and in a limited number of patients, suggest that MSCs could have a beneficial effect in cases of recurrent post-transplant FSGS resistant to conventional therapies. The mechanisms likely involve immunomodulatory, anti-inflammatory, and direct podocyte protection effects. However, larger controlled clinical studies are required to confirm these findings and establish the efficacy and safety of MSCs in this indication (**Table 6**).

10. Therapeutic plasma exchange, immunoadsorption, low density lipoprotein apheresis

The treatment of patients with FSGS recurrence after kidney transplantation is challenging and not well defined due to the lack of controlled studies both in adults and children which remains a topic of debate [172]. Various therapeutic options have been attempted, including apheresis procedures.

The pathophysiology of FSGS remains controversial, although it is believed to be caused by one or several circulating factors that target podocytes. Circulating plasma proteins of 22–150 kDa have a high affinity for galactose and supposedly form a complex with immunoglobulins. The main circulating factors involved are anti-nephrin antibodies, anti-UCH-1 antibodies, anti-CD40 antibodies, and cytokines such as CLCF-1, sUPAR, sCD40L, hemopexin, IL3, TNF-α, and BAFF [39–45, 49, 52, 73].

The participation of one or several circulating factors in FSGS has led to the use of various extracorporeal systems for treatment, such as plasma exchange (PE), immunoadsorption, and low-density lipoprotein (LDL-A) therapy [173].

For treatment monitoring, partial remission is defined as a > 50% reduction in proteinuria with respect to the initial value and ideally to <3.5 g/day and complete remission as proteinuria <0.5 g/day, with improvement in creatinine levels [174].

10.1 Therapeutic plasma exchange (TPE)

TPE is an extracorporeal purification technique that is performed by centrifugation or filtration. This last technique uses a high permeability membrane with a large pore size greater than 0.3 microns, allowing the separation of plasma and the elimination of medium and medium molecules with high molecular weight, such as cytokines and immunoglobulins, (**Figure 3**) [175].

The likelihood of achieving remission depends on the timing of TPE initiation. Early initiation of TPE in patients with rFSGS is associated with higher remission rates. A commonly used regimen includes 1.5 times plasma volume exchange for 3 consecutive days, followed by every other day for a total of 2 weeks or as improvement of proteinuria. The regimen is combined with standard anti-rejection medications, including rituximab, cyclosporine, mycophenolate mofetil, and corticosteroids [176].

A meta-analysis included results from six non-randomized studies involving 117 kidney transplant recipients and provides relatively valid evidence that

Drug	Mechanism of action in the podocyte
Corticosteroids	• Increase nephrin phosphorylation • Activate SGK1 and Src family kinases • Regulate podocin and nephrin expression through KLF15 factor • Downregulate caveolin-1 and TRPC6 • Downregulate CD80 expression • Stabilize synaptopodin by upregulating RhoA and downregulating RAC1 • Alter cytoskeleton organization
Calcineurin inhibitors (Cyclosporine A, Tacrolimus)	• Prevent cathepsin L-mediated synaptopodin degradation • Stabilize podocyte cytoskeleton by upregulating cofilin expression • Reduce intracellular calcium influx • Block mutant TRPC6 channels
Antimetabolites (mycophenolate mofetil)	• Attenuate urokinase receptor (uPAR) expression • Reduce podocyte apoptosis • Reduce RAC1 activation • Regulate expression of cell cycle proteins p27 and p21
mTOR inhibitors (sirolimus)	• Regulate podocyte size through mTORC1 • Moderate mTOR inhibition may have beneficial effects
Rituximab	• Binds to SMPDL-3b on podocytes • Regulates acid sphingomyelinase (ASMase) activity
SGLT2 inhibitors	• Reduce albuminuria and decrease the rate of eGFR decline
ACE inhibitors/ARBs	• Block the effects of the renin-angiotensin system on podocytes
Ofatumumab	• Binds to CD20 antigen on B lymphocytes (indirect effect on podocytes)
Abatacept/belatacept	• Potentially bind to B7–1 (CD80) on podocytes
Anti-TNFα	• Block the effects of TNFα on podocyte cytoskeleton and adhesion
Mesenchymal stem cells	• Paracrine effects promoting podocyte survival and function • Anti-inflammatory and immunomodulatory effects

Table 6.
Drugs and mechanisms of action in the podocyte.

implementation of TPE for rFSGS leads to disease remission and potentially protects against kidney allograft loss [177].

Recent consensus recommendations for TPE in rFSGS are:

We recommend immediate initial therapy of rFSGS with intensive plasmapheresis (1C).

We recommend against performing prophylactic plasmapheresis or rituximab before kidney transplantation (2C) [6].

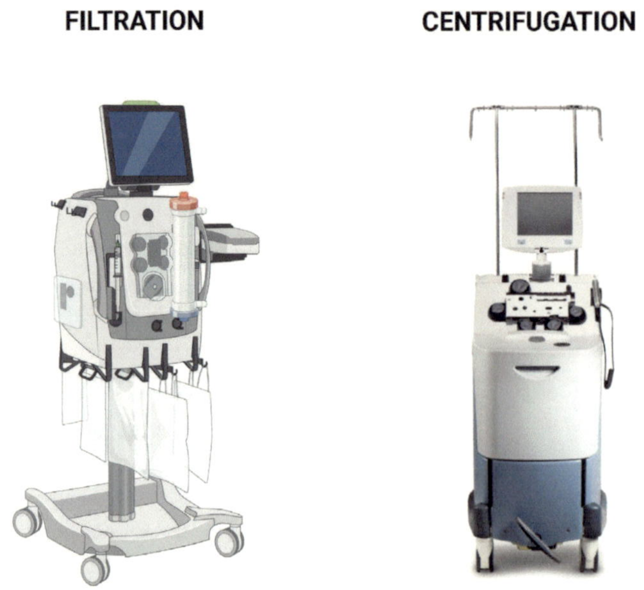

Figure 3.
Therapeutic plasma exchange techniques. Ref. [175].

Regarding the duration and interruption and number of procedures, different protocols have been proposed, one of them is to start with 3 TPE daily followed by at least 6 more TPE in the following 2 weeks, although other approaches have been reported.

Proteinuria is the key parameter to evaluate and monitor the response to treatment. The results with preventive treatment have not been consistent. Tapering of apheresis treatment should be decided on a case-by-case basis and is guided by the degree of proteinuria. The timing of clinical response is variable, and complete elimination of proteinuria may take several weeks to months. Some patients require long-term regimens of weekly or monthly TPE to prevent recurrence of proteinuria. There are no clinical or laboratory characteristics that predict the probability of success with TPE [6].

However, TPE induces a loss of coagulation factors responsible for side effects such as postoperative bleeding. Unlike TPE, immunoadsorption is a selective apheretic procedure. Dantal et al. [178] demonstrated a beneficial effect of IA therapy in adults with FSGS relapse after KTx (**Table 7**).

10.2 Immunoadsorption (IA)

Immunoadsorption is a semi-selective system that is beginning to gain ground in the treatment of FSGS. IA is a modification of PE in which circulating factors are selectively removed from separated plasma with the help of specific ligands on high-affinity absorption columns (**Figure 2**) [179, 180].

Immunoadsorption should be performed initially with 2.5 to 3 volumes of plasma and should be performed every day for 1 week, followed by every other day treatments for further 2 weeks and then twice a week for another 2 weeks (**Figure 4**) [6, 181, 182].

The procedure requires central venous access to ensure blood flow of 100–150 ml/min. The blood first passes through a plasma or cell separator that separates plasma from blood components. This separated plasma flows into a second machine containing the immunoadsorption columns.

Treatment phase	Frequency	Duration	Exchange volume
Initial	Daily for 3 consecutive days	3 days	1.5 times plasma volume
Intensive phase	Every other day	2 weeks	1.5 times plasma volume
Early maintenance	Three sessions per week	3 weeks	Not specified
Intermediate maintenance	Two sessions per week	3 weeks	Not specified
Late maintenance	One session per week	Until month 3	Not specified
Extended maintenance	Two sessions per month	Until month 5	Not specified
Final maintenance	One session per month	Until month 9	Not specified

Table 7.
Therapeutic plasma exchange (TPE) protocol for recurrent FSGS post-kidney transplantation [6].

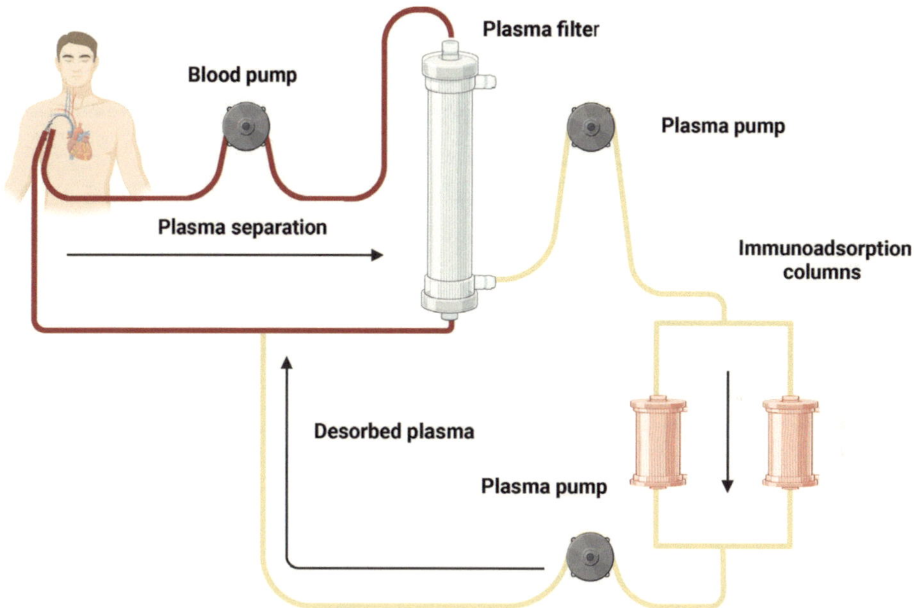

Figure 4.
Immunoadsorption technique [181].

The system uses two columns that function alternately – while plasma passes through one column, the second is regenerating. Once the active column becomes saturated, the flow switches to the second column while the first regenerates. This dual system allows continuous plasma treatment with no theoretical limit on the volume that can be treated. The columns contain a matrix with molecules (synthetic or organic) that bind to specific immunoglobulins. During the procedure, anticoagulation is required, typically with sodium citrate and intravenous calcium replacement, although heparin can also be used in combination with citrate.

Recent consensus recommendations for IA in rFSGS are:

We suggest that plasmapheresis or immunoadsorption be reinstituted in patients who respond successfully to initial sessions of plasmapheresis but then relapse (2C) [6].

Compared to TPE with IA, it is not necessary to substitute with albumin or plasma. In most cases, the hemodynamic tolerance of IA was much better than that of

PP. Furthermore, compared to TPE, coagulation factors are not lost with IA, limiting the risk of bleeding. However, after a few IA sessions, hypogammaglobulinemia can develop, which also occurs with the non-protein A anti-Ig affinity column and the protein A column [180, 183].

In this French AI cohort in pediatric post-transplant patients with FSGS recurrence, we reported the efficacy and safety of AI in 10 of 12 children, considering this as a therapeutic option in FSGS recurrence after KTx, and it is an alternative therapy to TPE for its more selective performance. Additional follow-up will be required to determine the long-term prognosis of these patients [172].

10.3 Low density lipoprotein apheresis

Muso et al. [183] conducted a multicenter prospective observational survey on the long-term effect of flow density lipid (LDL) apheresis in 54 adults with drug-resistant nephrotic syndrome (POLARIS study). Of the 44 subjects (followed for 2 years),

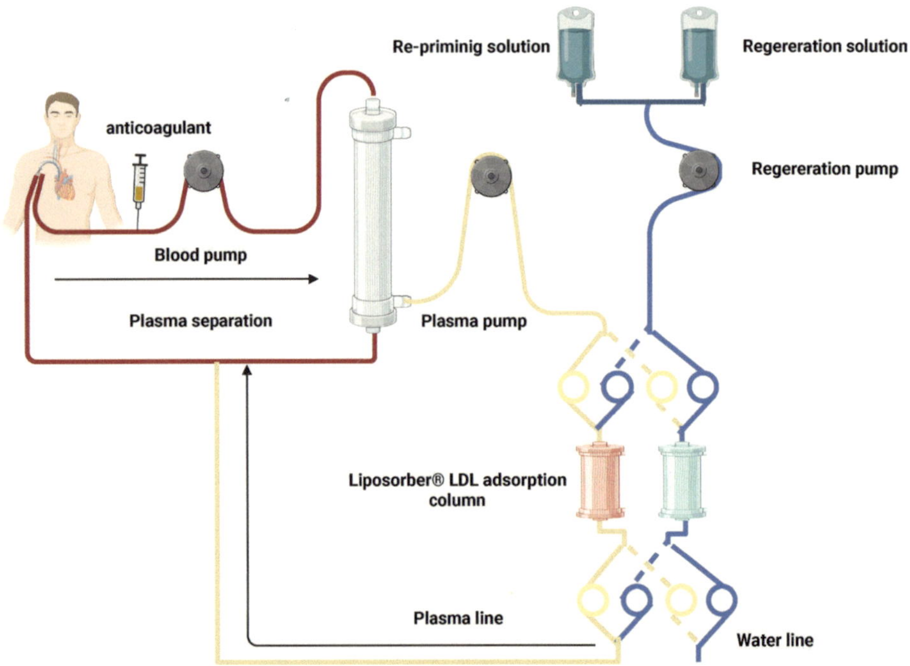

Figure 5.
*Low density lipoprotein apheresis technique [185]. Blood is drawn from the patient through venous access, and heparin is added as an anticoagulant. Plasma is separated from cellular elements using a membrane filter. The separated plasma passes through columns containing cellulose beads coated with dextran sulfate. Apo B, which has a positive charge, binds non-covalently to negatively charged dextran sulfate. Thus, the column selectively adsorbs LDL, VLDL and Lp(a), but not HDL. The system uses two dextran sulfate columns that are used alternately to remove atherogenic lipoproteins. The columns are automatically cleaned and regenerated by the system so that there is always a column ready. This allows continuous operation with large volumes without oversaturation. In this protocol, each patient received a minimum of 9 weeks of LDL-A treatment using an exchange volume of 60 ml/kg. In the first 3 weeks, patients received 2 to 3 weekly sessions of LDL-A. In the remaining weeks until discontinuation, patients underwent LDL-A weekly. After the first 3 weeks of LDL-A treatment, patients received pulse doses of 10 to 20 mg/kg IV methylprednisolone with a maximum single dose of 1 g [185]. After completion of LDL-A, individual treatment centers tapered oral prednisone at their discretion. While the protocol aimed to define the duration of LDL-A at 9 weeks, some centers chose to continue therapy for longer periods. The use of LDL-A does not require blood preparation [185]. More studies will be required to determine the long-term prognosis of these patients (***Table 8***).*

Week	LDL-A sessions per week	Steroids
1	2–3	S
2	2–3	S
3	2–3	S
4	1	S
5	1	S
6	1	S
7	1	S
8	1	S
9	1	S

Table 8.
LDL-apheresis treatment protocol [185].

21 (47.7%) showed remission of nephrotic syndrome based on urinary protein (UP) levels of <1.0 g/day. The UP level immediately after LDL-A and the improvement rates of UP, serum albumin, serum creatinine, eGFR, and total and LDL cholesterol after treatment significantly affected the results.

Raina et al. [184] reported on 11 pediatric patients with FSGS who were resistant to steroids and cyclosporine and where apheresis (LDL apheresis) induced a CR of 45% and a PR of 18%; mean proteinuria decreased from 9.7 ± 2.5 to 1 ± 0.5 g/L ($p < 0.05$) (**Figure** 5).

11. Conclusions

Recurrent FSGS post-kidney transplantation remains a significant clinical challenge, characterized by high recurrence rates and a complex pathogenesis involving multiple circulating factors harmful to podocytes. Despite advances in understanding the underlying molecular mechanisms, definitive biomarkers for its prediction or early diagnosis are still lacking. Current therapeutic management, primarily based on plasmapheresis and immunosuppression, shows variable and unpredictable results, which has driven research into new targeted therapies such as monoclonal antibodies and SGLT2 inhibitors. Although these new therapeutic options, including cellular therapies, show promising results in some patients, multicenter controlled and randomized studies are required to establish their efficacy and optimal treatment protocols. In this context, an individualized and multidisciplinary treatment approach emerges as the most appropriate strategy at present. The field of recurrent FSGS post-transplantation continues to be an active area of research, with multiple questions yet to be resolved, especially regarding prevention, early diagnosis, and effective treatment. It is anticipated that ongoing evolution in the understanding of underlying molecular mechanisms will lead to the development of more targeted and effective therapies in the future.

Author details

Maiko Alejandro Tavera Díaz[1*], David Andrés Ballesteros Castro[2], Omar Lafuente Covarrubias[3], Alison Vannia Nava Rojas[1] and Israel Danny Rivas Salazar[3]

1 Univalle Hospital, Cochabamba, Bolivia

2 San José University Hospital, Popayán, Popayan, Colombia

3 Caja Nacional de Salud, Cochabamba, Bolivia

*Address all correspondence to: taveradiaz@gmail.com

References

[1] D'Agati VD, Fogo AB, Bruijn JA, Jennette JC. Pathologic classification of focal segmental glomerulosclerosis: A working proposal. American Journal of Kidney Diseases. 2004;**43**(2):368-382. DOI: 10.1053/j.ajkd.2003.10.024

[2] Kitiyakara C, Kopp JB, Eggers P. Trends in the epidemiology of focal segmental glomerulosclerosis. Seminars in Nephrology. 2003;**23**(2):172-182. DOI: 10.1053/snep.2003.50025

[3] Johansen KL, Chertow GM, Gilbertson DT, Ishani A, Israni A, Ku E, et al. US renal data system 2022 Annual Data Report: Epidemiology of kidney disease in the United States. American Journal of Kidney Diseases. 2023;**81**(3 Suppl. 1):A8-A11. DOI: 10.1053/j.ajkd.2022.12.001

[4] McDonnell T, Storrar J, Chinnadurai R, Heal C, Chrysochou C, Ritchie J, et al. The epidemiology of primary FSGS including cluster analysis over a 20-year period. BMC Nephrology. 2023;**24**(1):365. DOI: 10.1186/s12882-023-03405-w

[5] Rovin BH, Adler SG, Barratt J, Bridoux F, Burdge KA, Chan TM, et al. KDIGO 2021 clinical practice guideline for the management of glomerular diseases. Kidney International. 2021;**100**(4):S1-S276. DOI: 10.1016/j.kint.2021.05.021

[6] Raina R, Jothi S, Haffner D, Somers M, Filler G, Vasistha P, et al. Post-transplant recurrence of focal segmental glomerular sclerosis: Consensus statements. Kidney International. 2024;**105**(3):450-463. DOI: 10.1016/j.kint.2023.10.017. Epub 2023 Dec 22

[7] Ichimura K, Miyazaki N, Sadayama S, Murata K, Koike M, Nakamura K, et al. Three-dimensional architecture of podocytes revealed by block-face scanning electron microscopy. Scientific Reports. 2015;**5**:8993. DOI: 10.1038/srep08993

[8] Blaine J, Dylewski J. Regulation of the actin cytoskeleton in Podocytes. Cells. 2020;**9**(7):1700. DOI: 10.3390/cells9071700

[9] Pozzi A, Jarad G, Moeckel GW, Coffa S, Zhang X, Gewin L, et al. Beta1 integrin expression by podocytes is required to maintain glomerular structural integrity. Developmental Biology. 2008;**316**(2):288-301. DOI: 10.1016/j.ydbio.2008.01.022. Epub 2008 Jan 31

[10] Martin CE, Jones N. Nephrin signaling in the Podocyte: An updated view of signal regulation at the slit diaphragm and beyond. Frontiers in Endocrinology (Lausanne). 2018;**9**:302. DOI: 10.3389/fendo.2018.00302

[11] Kerjaschki D. Caught flat-footed: Podocyte damage and the molecular bases of focal glomerulosclerosis. The Journal of Clinical Investigation. 2001;**108**(11):1583-1587. DOI: 10.1172/JCI14629

[12] Perico L, Conti S, Benigni A, Remuzzi G. Podocyte-actin dynamics in health and disease. Nature Reviews. Nephrology. 2016;**12**(11):692-710. DOI: 10.1038/nrneph.2016.127. Epub 2016 Aug 30

[13] Ahmadian E, Eftekhari A, Atakishizada S, Valiyeva M, Ardalan M, Khalilov R, et al. Podocytopathy: The role of actin cytoskeleton. Biomedicine & Pharmacotherapy. 2022;**156**:113920. DOI: 10.1016/j.biopha.2022.113920. Epub 2022 Oct 27

[14] Sever S. Role of actin cytoskeleton in podocytes. Pediatric Nephrology. 2021;**36**(9):2607-2614. DOI: 10.1007/s00467-020-04812-z. Epub 2020 Nov 13

[15] Bai J, Zhang T, Wang Y, Cao J, Duan Z, Ji L, et al. Incidence and risk factors for recurrent focal segmental glomerulosclerosis after kidney transplantation: A meta-analysis. Renal Failure. 2023;**45**(1):2201341. DOI: 10.1080/0886022X.2023.2201341

[16] Uffing A, Pérez-Sáez MJ, Mazzali M, Manfro RC, Bauer AC, de Sottomaior DF, et al. Recurrence of FSGS after kidney transplantation in adults. Clinical Journal of the American Society of Nephrology. 2020;**15**(2):247-256. DOI: 10.2215/CJN.08970719. Epub 2020 Jan 23

[17] Abbott KC, Sawyers ES, Oliver JD 3rd, Ko CW, Kirk AD, Welch PG, et al. Graft loss due to recurrent focal segmental glomerulosclerosis in renal transplant recipients in the United States. American Journal of Kidney Diseases. 2001;**37**(2):366-373. DOI: 10.1053/ajkd.2001.21311

[18] Francis A, Trnka P, McTaggart SJ. Long-term outcome of kidney transplantation in recipients with focal segmental Glomerulosclerosis. Clinical Journal of the American Society of Nephrology. 2016;**11**(11):2041-2046. DOI: 10.2215/CJN.03060316. Epub 2016 Oct 20

[19] Huang K, Ferris ME, Andreoni KA, Gipson DS. The differential effect of race among pediatric kidney transplant recipients with focal segmental glomerulosclerosis. American Journal of Kidney Diseases. 2004;**43**(6):1082-1090. DOI: 10.1053/j.ajkd.2004.03.017

[20] Schachter ME, Monahan M, Radhakrishnan J, et al. Recurrent focal segmental glomerulosclerosis in the renal allograft: Single center experience in the era of modern immunosuppression. Clinical Nephrology. 2010;**74**(3):173-181

[21] Kim SJ, Ha J, Jung IM, et al. Recurrent focal segmental glomerulosclerosis following renal transplantation in Korean pediatric patients. Pediatric Transplantation. 2001;**5**(2):105-111

[22] Fujisawa M, Iijima K, Ishimura T, et al. Long-term outcome of focal segmental glomerulosclerosis after Japanese pediatric renal transplantation. Pediatric Nephrology. 2002;**17**(3):165-168

[23] Baum MA, Stablein DM, Panzarino VM, Tejani A, Harmon WE, Alexander SR. Loss of living donor renal allograft survival advantage in children with focal segmental glomerulosclerosis. Kidney International. 2001;**59**(1):328-333. DOI: 10.1046/j.1523-1755.2001.00494.x

[24] Briganti EM, Russ GR, McNeil JJ, Atkins RC, Chadban SJ. Risk of renal allograft loss from recurrent glomerulonephritis. The New England Journal of Medicine. 2002;**347**(2):103-109. DOI: 10.1056/NEJMoa013036

[25] Shalhoub RJ. Pathogenesis of lipoid nephrosis: A disorder of T-cell function. Lancet. 1974;**2**(7880):556-560. DOI: 10.1016/s0140-6736(74)91880-7

[26] Frank C, Herrmann M, Fernandez S, et al. Dominant T cells in idiopathic nephrotic syndrome of childhood. Kidney International. 2000;**57**(2):510-517

[27] Baris HE, Baris S, Karakoc-Aydiner E, et al. The effect of systemic corticosteroids on the innate and adaptive immune system in children with steroid responsive nephrotic syndrome. European Journal of Pediatrics. 2016;**175**(8):1073-1082

[28] Casiraghi F, Todeschini M, Podestà MA, et al. Immunophenotypic alterations in adult patients with steroid-dependent and frequently relapsing nephrotic syndrome. International Journal of Molecular Sciences. 2023;**24**(9):7687. Published 2023 Apr 22. DOI: 10.3390/ijms24097687

[29] Boumediene A, Vachin P, Sendeyo K, et al. NEPHRUTIX: A randomized, double-blind, placebo vs rituximab-controlled trial assessing T-cell subset changes in minimal change nephrotic syndrome. Journal of Autoimmunity. 2018;**88**:91-102. DOI: 10.1016/j.jaut.2017.10.006

[30] Chan CY, Liu ID, Resontoc LP, et al. T lymphocyte activation markers as predictors of responsiveness to rituximab among patients with FSGS. Clinical Journal of the American Society of Nephrology. 2016;**11**(8):1360-1368. DOI: 10.2215/CJN.11941115

[31] Wang L, Li Q, Wang L, Li C, Yang H, Wang X, et al. The role of Th17/IL-17 in the pathogenesis of primary nephrotic syndrome in children. Kidney & Blood Pressure Research. 2013;**37**(4-5):332-345. DOI: 10.1159/000350161. Epub 2013 Sep 23

[32] Ling C, Wang X, Chen Z, Fan J, Meng Q, Zhou N, et al. Altered B-lymphocyte homeostasis in idiopathic nephrotic syndrome. Frontiers in Pediatrics. 2019;7:377. DOI: 10.3389/fped.2019.00377

[33] Ling C, Chen Z, Fan J, Sun Q, Wang X, Hua L, et al. Decreased circulating transitional B-cell to memory B-cell ratio is a risk factor for relapse in children with steroid-sensitive nephrotic syndrome. Nephron. 2021;**145**(2):107-112. DOI: 10.1159/000511319. Epub 2020 Dec 22

[34] Anis S, Ahmed E, Muzaffar R, Rizv SAH. T and B cells immunophenotypes in blood and urine of patients with focal segmental glomerulosclerosis in relation to disease severity. Clinical Practice. 2018;**15**(5):811-819. DOI: 10.4172/clinical-practice.1000414

[35] Oniszczuk J, Beldi-Ferchiou A, Audureau E, Azzaoui I, Molinier-Frenkel V, Frontera V, et al. Circulating plasmablasts and high level of BAFF are hallmarks of minimal change nephrotic syndrome in adults. Nephrology, Dialysis, Transplantation. 2021;**36**(4):609-617. DOI: 10.1093/ndt/gfaa279

[36] Kalled SL. The role of BAFF in immune function and implications for autoimmunity. Immunological Reviews. 2005;**204**:43-54. DOI: 10.1111/j.0105-2896.2005.00219.x

[37] Alderson MR, Armitage RJ, Tough TW, Strockbine L, Fanslow WC, Spriggs MK. CD40 expression by human monocytes: Regulation by cytokines and activation of monocytes by the ligand for CD40. The Journal of Experimental Medicine. 1993;**178**(2):669-674. DOI: 10.1084/jem.178.2.669

[38] Doublier S, Zennaro C, Musante L, Spatola T, Candiano G, Bruschi M, et al. Soluble CD40 ligand directly alters glomerular permeability and may act as a circulating permeability factor in FSGS. PLoS One. 2017;**12**(11):e0188045. DOI: 10.1371/journal.pone.0188045

[39] Shirai Y, Miura K, Ishizuka K, Ando T, Kanda S, Hashimoto J, et al. A multi-institutional study found a possible role of anti-nephrin antibodies in post-transplant focal segmental glomerulosclerosis recurrence. Kidney International. 2024;**105**(3):608-617. DOI: 10.1016/j.kint.2023.11.022. Epub 2023 Dec 16

[40] Hengel FE, Dehde S, Lassé M, Zahner G, Seifert L, Schnarre A, et al.

Autoantibodies targeting nephrin in podocytopathies. The New England Journal of Medicine. 1 Aug 2024;**391**(5):422-433. DOI: 10.1056/NEJMoa2314471

[41] Reichelt J, Sachs W, Frömbling S, Fehlert J, Studencka-Turski M, Betz A, et al. Non-functional ubiquitin C-terminal hydrolase L1 drives podocyte injury through impairing proteasomes in autoimmune glomerulonephritis. Nature Communications. 2023;**14**(1):2114. DOI: 10.1038/s41467-023-37836-8. Erratum in: Nat Commun. 2023 Apr 28;14(1):2453. doi: 10.1038/s41467-023-38206-0

[42] Jamin A, Berthelot L, Couderc A, Chemouny JM, Boedec E, Dehoux L, et al. Autoantibodies against podocytic UCHL1 are associated with idiopathic nephrotic syndrome relapses and induce proteinuria in mice. Journal of Autoimmunity. 2018;**89**:149-161. DOI: 10.1016/j.jaut.2017.12.014. Epub 2018 Jan 4

[43] Karnell JL, Rieder SA, Ettinger R, Kolbeck R. Targeting the CD40-CD40L pathway in autoimmune diseases: Humoral immunity and beyond. Advanced Drug Delivery Reviews. 2019;**141**:92-103. DOI: 10.1016/j.addr.2018.12.005

[44] Chebotareva N, Cao V, Vinogradov A, Alentov I, Sergeeva N, Kononikhin A, et al. Preliminary study of anti-CD40 and ubiquitin proteasome antibodies in primary podocytopaties. Frontiers in Medicine (Lausanne). 2023;**10**:1189017. DOI: 10.3389/fmed.2023.1189017

[45] Savin VJ, Sharma M, Zhou J, Gennochi D, Fields T, Sharma R, et al. Renal and hematological effects of CLCF-1, a B-cell-stimulating cytokine of the IL-6 family. Journal of Immunology Research. 2015;**2015**:714964. DOI: 10.1155/2015/714964. Epub 2015 Jun 4

[46] Vlotides G, Zitzmann K, Stalla GK, Auernhammer CJ. Novel neurotrophin-1/B cell-stimulating factor-3 (NNT-1/BSF-3)/cardiotrophin-like cytokine (CLC)–A novel gp130 cytokine with pleiotropic functions. Cytokine & Growth Factor Reviews. 2004;**15**(5):325-336. DOI: 10.1016/j.cytogfr.2004.04.002

[47] Sharma M, Zhou J, Gauchat JF, Sharma R, McCarthy ET, Srivastava T, et al. Janus kinase 2/signal transducer and activator of transcription 3 inhibitors attenuate the effect of cardiotrophin-like cytokine factor 1 and human focal segmental glomerulosclerosis serum on glomerular filtration barrier. Translational Research. 2015;**166**(4):384-398. DOI: 10.1016/j.trsl.2015.03.002. Epub 2015 Mar 16

[48] Wei C, Möller CC, Altintas MM, Li J, Schwarz K, Zacchigna S, et al. Modification of kidney barrier function by the urokinase receptor. Nature Medicine. 2008;**14**(1):55-63. DOI: 10.1038/nm1696. Epub 2007 Dec 16

[49] Wei C, El Hindi S, Li J, Fornoni A, Goes N, Sageshima J, et al. Circulating urokinase receptor as a cause of focal segmental glomerulosclerosis. Nature Medicine. 2011;**17**(8):952-960. DOI: 10.1038/nm.2411

[50] Maas RJ, Deegens JK, Wetzels JF. Serum suPAR in patients with FSGS: Trash or treasure? Pediatric Nephrology. 2013;**28**(7):1041-1048. DOI: 10.1007/s00467-013-2452-5. Epub 2013 Mar 21

[51] Bock ME, Price HE, Gallon L, Langman CB. Serum soluble urokinase-type plasminogen activator receptor levels and idiopathic FSGS in children: A single-center report. Clinical Journal of the American Society of Nephrology.

2013;**8**(8):1304-1311. DOI: 10.2215/CJN.07680712. Epub 2013 Apr 25

[52] Tolosano E, Altruda F. Hemopexin: Structure, function, and regulation. DNA and Cell Biology. 2002;**21**(4):297-306. DOI: 10.1089/104454902753759717

[53] Cheung PK, Klok PA, Baller JF, Bakker WW. Induction of experimental proteinuria in vivo following infusion of human plasma hemopexin. Kidney International. 2000;**57**(4):1512-1520. DOI: 10.1046/j.1523-1755.2000.00996.x

[54] Lennon R, Singh A, Welsh GI, Coward RJ, Satchell S, Ni L, et al. Hemopexin induces nephrin-dependent reorganization of the actin cytoskeleton in podocytes. Journal of the American Society of Nephrology : JASN. 2008;**19**(11):2140-2149. DOI: 10.1681/ASN.2007080940. Epub 2008 Aug 27

[55] Kimata H, Fujimoto M, Furusho K. Involvement of interleukin (IL)-13, but not IL-4, in spontaneous IgE and IgG4 production in nephrotic syndrome. European Journal of Immunology. 1995;**25**(6):1497-1501. DOI: 10.1002/eji.1830250604

[56] Lai KW, Wei CL, Tan LK, Tan PH, Chiang GS, Lee CG, et al. Overexpression of interleukin-13 induces minimal-change-like nephropathy in rats. Journal of the American Society of Nephrology: JASN. 2007;**18**(5):1476-1485. DOI: 10.1681/ASN.2006070710. Epub 2007 Apr 11

[57] Yap HK, Cheung W, Murugasu B, Sim SK, Seah CC, Jordan SC. Th1 and Th2 cytokine mRNA profiles in childhood nephrotic syndrome: Evidence for increased IL-13 mRNA expression in relapse. Journal of the American Society of Nephrology : JASN. 1999;**10**(3):529-537. DOI: 10.1681/ASN.V103529

[58] Otalora L, Chavez E, Watford D, Tueros L, Correa M, Nair V, et al. Identification of glomerular and podocyte-specific genes and pathways activated by sera of patients with focal segmental glomerulosclerosis. PLoS One. 2019;**14**(10):e0222948. DOI: 10.1371/journal.pone.0222948

[59] Chung CF, Kitzler T, Kachurina N, Pessina K, Babayeva S, Bitzan M, et al. Intrinsic tumor necrosis factor-α pathway is activated in a subset of patients with focal segmental glomerulosclerosis. PLoS One. 2019;**14**(5):e0216426. DOI: 10.1371/journal.pone.0216426

[60] Bossen C, Schneider P. BAFF, APRIL and their receptors: Structure, function and signaling. Seminars in Immunology. 2006;**18**(5):263-275. DOI: 10.1016/j.smim.2006.04.006. Epub 2006 Aug 17

[61] Hoffman W, Lakkis FG, Chalasani G. B cells, antibodies, and more. Clinical Journal of the American Society of Nephrology. 2016;**11**(1):137-154. DOI: 10.2215/CJN.09430915. Epub 2015 Dec 23

[62] Lahiri A, Pochard P, Le Pottier L, Tobón GJ, Bendaoud B, Youinou P, et al. The complexity of the BAFF TNF-family members: Implications for autoimmunity. Journal of Autoimmunity. 2012;**39**:189-198. DOI: 10.1016/j.jaut.2012.05.009

[63] Forero-Delgadillo J, Ochoa V, Restrepo JM, Torres-Canchala L, Nieto-Aristizábal I, Ruiz-Ordoñez I, et al. B-cell activating factor (BAFF) and its receptors' expression in pediatric nephrotic syndrome is associated with worse prognosis. PLoS One. 2022;**17**(11):e0277800. DOI: 10.1371/journal.pone.0277800

[64] Latt KZ, Heymann J, Jessee JH, Rosenberg AZ, Berthier CC, Arazi A, et al. Urine single-cell RNA sequencing in focal segmental glomerulosclerosis

reveals inflammatory signatures. Kidney International Reports. 2021;**7**(2):289-304. DOI: 10.1016/j.ekir.2021.11.005

[65] Savin VJ, Sharma R, Sharma M, McCarthy ET, Swan SK, Ellis E, et al. Circulating factor associated with increased glomerular permeability to albumin in recurrent focal segmental glomerulosclerosis. The New England Journal of Medicine. 1996;**334**(14):878-883. DOI: 10.1056/NEJM199604043341402

[66] Gallon L, Leventhal J, Skaro A, Kanwar Y, Alvarado A. Resolution of recurrent focal segmental glomerulosclerosisafterretransplantation. The New England Journal of Medicine. 2012;**366**(17):1648-1649. DOI: 10.1056/NEJMc1202500

[67] Salfi G, Casiraghi F, Remuzzi G. Current understanding of the molecular mechanisms of circulating permeability factor in focal segmental glomerulosclerosis. Frontiers in Immunology. 2023;**14**:1247606. DOI: 10.3389/fimmu.2023.1247606

[68] Watts AJB, Keller KH, Lerner G, Rosales I, Collins AB, Sekulic M, et al. Discovery of autoantibodies targeting nephrin in minimal change disease supports a novel autoimmune Etiology. Journal of the American Society of Nephrology : JASN. 2022;**33**(1):238-252. DOI: 10.1681/ASN.2021060794. Epub 2021 Nov 3

[69] Radón V, Czesla M, Reichelt J, Fehlert J, Hammel A, Rosendahl A, et al. Ubiquitin C-terminal hydrolase L1 is required for regulated protein degradation through the ubiquitin proteasome system in kidney. Kidney International. 2018;**93**(1):110-127. DOI: 10.1016/j.kint.2017.05.016. Epub 2017 Jul 26

[70] Delville M, Sigdel TK, Wei C, Li J, Hsieh SC, Fornoni A, et al. A circulating antibody panel for pretransplant prediction of FSGS recurrence after kidney transplantation. Science Translational Medicine. 2014;**6**(256):256ra136. DOI: 10.1126/scitranslmed.3008538

[71] Rashmi P, Sigdel TK, Rychkov D, Damm I, Da Silva AA, Vincenti F, et al. Perturbations in podocyte transcriptome and biological pathways induced by FSGS associated circulating factors. Annals of Translational Medicine. 2023;**11**(9):315. DOI: 10.21037/atm-22-3670. Epub 2023 May 4

[72] McCarthy ET, Sharma M, Savin VJ. Circulating permeability factors in idiopathic nephrotic syndrome and focal segmental glomerulosclerosis. Clinical Journal of the American Society of Nephrology. 2010;**5**(11):2115-2121. DOI: 10.2215/CJN.03800609. Epub 2010 Oct 21

[73] De Smet E, Rioux J-P, Ammann H, Deziel C, Querin S. FSGS permeability factor-associated nephrotic syndrome: Remission after oral galactose therapy. Nephrology, Dialysis, Transplantation. 2009;**24**:2938-2940. DOI: 10.1093/ndt/gfp278

[74] Sgambat K, Banks M, Moudgil A. Effect of galactose on glomerular permeability and proteinuria in steroid-resistant nephrotic syndrome. Pediatric Nephrology. 2013;**28**(11):2131-2135. DOI: 10.1007/s00467-013-2539-z. Epub 2013 Jun 22

[75] Thunø M, Macho B, Eugen-Olsen J. suPAR: The molecular crystal ball. Disease Markers. 2009;**27**(3):157-172. DOI: 10.3233/DMA-2009-0657

[76] Kapojos JJ, van den Berg A, van Goor H, te Loo MW, Poelstra K, Borghuis T, et al. Production of hemopexin by TNF-alpha stimulated

human mesangial cells. Kidney International. 2003;**63**(5):1681-1686. DOI: 10.1046/j.1523-1755.2003.00907.x

[77] Pukajło-Marczyk A, Zwolińska D. Involvement of hemopexin in the pathogenesis of proteinuria in children with idiopathic nephrotic syndrome. Journal of Clinical Medicine. 2021;**10**(14):3160. DOI: 10.3390/jcm10143160

[78] Chebotareva NV, Vinogradov A, Brzhozovskiy AG, Kashirina DN, Indeykina MI, Bugrova AE, et al. Potential urine proteomic biomarkers for focal segmental glomerulosclerosis and minimal change disease. International Journal of Molecular Sciences. 2022;**23**(20):12607. DOI: 10.3390/ijms232012607

[79] Stangou M, Spartalis M, Daikidou D-V, Kouloukourgiotou T, Sampani E, Lambropoulou I-T, et al. Impact of Th1 and Th2 cytokines in the progression of idiopathic nephrotic syndrome due to focal segmental glomerulosclerosis and minimal change disease. Journal of Nephropathology. 2016;**6**:187-195. DOI: 10.15171/jnp.2017.32

[80] Prossnitz ER, Sklar LA. Chemotactic peptide/complement receptors. In: Encyclopedia of Biological Chemistry. 2nd ed. Academic Press; 2013. pp. 493-497. DOI: 10.1016/B978-0-12-378630-2.00342-X

[81] Joy MS, Gipson DS, Powell L, MacHardy J, Jennette JC, Vento S, et al. Phase 1 trial of adalimumab in focal segmental glomerulosclerosis (FSGS): II. Report of the FONT (novel therapies for resistant FSGS) study group. American Journal of Kidney Diseases. 2010;**55**(1):50-60. DOI: 10.1053/j.ajkd.2009.08.019. Epub 2009 Nov 22

[82] Cancro MP, D'Cruz DP, Khamashta MA. The role of B lymphocyte stimulator (BLyS) in systemic lupus erythematosus. The Journal of Clinical Investigation. 2009;**119**(5):1066-1073. DOI: 10.1172/JCI38010. Epub 2009 May 1

[83] Scapini P, Nardelli B, Nadali G, Calzetti F, Pizzolo G, Montecucco C, et al. G-CSF-stimulated neutrophils are a prominent source of functional BLyS. The Journal of Experimental Medicine. 2003;**197**(3):297-302. DOI: 10.1084/jem.20021343

[84] Paiano J, Harland M, Strainic MG, Nedrud J, Hussain W, Medof ME. Follicular B2 cell activation and class switch recombination depend on autocrine C3ar1/C5ar1 signaling in B2 cells. Journal of Immunology. 2019;**203**:379-388. DOI: 10.4049/jimmunol.1900276

[85] Sciascia S, Radin M, Yazdany J, Levy RA, Roccatello D, Dall'Era M, et al. Efficacy of belimumab on renal outcomes in patients with systemic lupus erythematosus: A systematic review. Autoimmunity Reviews. 2017;**16**(3):287-293. DOI: 10.1016/j.autrev.2017.01.010. Epub 2017 Jan 29

[86] Infante B, Rossini M, Leo S, Troise D, Netti GS, Ranieri E, et al. Recurrent glomerulonephritis after renal transplantation: The clinical problem. International Journal of Molecular Sciences. 19 Aug 2020;**21**(17):5954. DOI: 10.3390/ijms21175954

[87] Radha S, Afroz T, Prasad CR, Sridhar G, Rajaram KG, Reddy S. Focal segmental glomerulosclerosis in renal allografts: Is it possible to diagnose the etiology? Indian Journal of Nephrology [Internet]. 2015;**25**(2):82-85. DOI: 10.4103/0971-4065.137173

[88] English M, Hawryluk E, Krupnick R, Kumar MSA, Schwartz J. The symptoms

and impact of recurrent focal segmental glomerulosclerosis in kidney transplant recipients: A conceptual model of the patient experience. Advances in Therapy [Internet]. 2019;**36**(12):3390-3408. DOI: 10.1007/s12325-019-01110-5

[89] Taneda S, Honda K, Koike J, Ito N, Ishida H, Takagi T, et al. Clinicopathological differences in focal segmental glomerulosclerosis depending on the accompanying pathophysiological conditions in renal allografts. Virchows Archiv [Internet]. 2023;**483**(6):809-819. DOI: 10.1007/s00428-023-03703-6

[90] Tejani A, Stablein DH. Recurrence of focal segmental glomerulosclerosis posttransplantation: A special report of the north American Pediatric Renal Transplant Cooperative Study. Journal of the American Society of Nephrology : JASN [Internet]. 1992;**2**(12 Suppl.):S258-S263. DOI: 10.1681/ASN.V212s258

[91] Fuentes GMC, Meseguer CG, Carrion AP, Hijosa MM, Garcia-Pose A, Melgar AA, et al. Long-term outcome of focal segmental glomerulosclerosis after pediatric renal transplantation. Pediatric Nephrology [Internet]. 2010;**25**(3):529-534. DOI: 10.1007/s00467-009-1361-0

[92] Alasfar S, Matar D, Montgomery RA, Desai N, Lonze B, Vujjini V, et al. Rituximab and therapeutic plasma exchange in recurrent focal segmental glomerulosclerosis postkidney transplantation. Transplantation. 2018;**102**(3):e115-e120. DOI: 10.1097/TP.0000000000002008

[93] Hickson LJ, Gera M, Amer H, Iqbal CW, Moore TB, Milliner DS, et al. Kidney transplantation for primary focal segmental glomerulosclerosis: Outcomes and response to therapy for recurrence. Transplantation [Internet]. 2009;**87**(8):1232-1239. DOI: 10.1097/TP.0b013e31819f12be

[94] Scalamogna M, Ginevri F. Prediction and treatment of recurrent focal segmental glomerulosclerosis after renal transplantation in children. American Journal of Kidney Diseases. Dec 1999;**34**(6):1048-1055. DOI: 10.1016/S0272-6386(99)70010-7

[95] Couser W. Recurrent glomerulonephritis in the renal allograft: An update of selected areas. Experimental and Clinical Transplantation [Internet]. 2005;**3**(1):283-288. Available from: https://www.ncbi.nlm.nih.gov/pubmed/15989671

[96] Choi KH, Kim SI, Yoon SY, Kim JH, Kang SW, Ha SK, et al. Long-term outcome of kidney transplantation in adult recipients with focal segmental glomerulosclerosis. Yonsei Medical Journal [Internet]. 2001;**42**(2):209-214. Available from: http://eymj.org/Synapse/Data/PDFData/0069YMJ/ymj-42-209.pdf

[97] Crosson JT. Focal segmental glomerulosclerosis and renal transplantation. Transplantation Proceedings [Internet]. 2007;**39**(3):737-743. DOI: 10.1016/j.transproceed.2007.02.010

[98] Uffing A, Pérez-Sáez MJ, La Manna G, Comai G, Fischman C, Farouk S, et al. A large, international study on post-transplant glomerular diseases: The TANGO project. BMC Nephrology [Internet]. 2018;**19**(1):229. DOI: 10.1186/s12882-018-1025-z

[99] Ponticelli C. Recurrence of focal segmental glomerular sclerosis (FSGS) after renal transplantation. Nephrology, Dialysis, Transplantation. 2010;**25**(1):25-31. DOI: 10.1093/ndt/gfp538

[100] Kwon HE, Kim YH, Lee SA, Lee JJ, Ko Y, Shin S, et al. Post-operative

recurrence of focal segmental glomerulosclerosis according to pre-transplant treatment after kidney transplantation. BMC Nephrology [Internet]. 2023;**24**(1):53. DOI: 10.1186/s12882-023-03098-1

[101] Campise M, Favi E, Messa P. Clinical outcomes of prophylactic and therapeutic plasmapheresis in adult deceased-donor kidney transplant recipients with primary focal segmental glomerulosclerosis. Experimental and Clinical Transplantation [Internet]. 2019;**17**(4):461-469. DOI: 10.6002/ect.2018.0106

[102] Gohh RY, Yango AF, Morrissey PE, Monaco AP, Gautam A, Sharma M, et al. Preemptive plasmapheresis and recurrence of FSGS in high-risk renal transplant recipients. American Journal of Transplantation. 2005;**5**(12):2907-2912. DOI: 10.1111/j.1600-6143.2005.01112.x

[103] Ohta T, Kawaguchi H, Hattori M, Komatsu Y, Akioka Y, Nagata M, et al. Effect of pre-and postoperative plasmapheresis on posttransplant recurrence of focal segmental glomerulosclerosis in children. Transplantation. 2001;**71**(5):628-633. DOI: 10.1097/00007890-200103150-00008

[104] Boonpheng B, Hansrivijit P, Thongprayoon C, Mao SA, Vaitla PK, Bathini T, et al. Rituximab or plasmapheresis for prevention of recurrent focal segmental glomerulosclerosis after kidney transplantation: A systematic review and meta-analysis. World Journal of Transplantation. 2021;**11**(7):303-319. DOI: 10.5500/wjt.v11.i7.303

[105] Salvadori M, Tsalouchos A. How immunosuppressive drugs may directly target podocytes in glomerular diseases. Pediatric Nephrology. 2022;**37**(7):1431-1441. DOI: 10.1007/s00467-021-05196-4. Epub 2021 Jul 9

[106] Mallipattu SK, Liu R, Zheng F, Narla G, Ma'ayan A, Dikman S, et al. Kruppel-like factor 15 (KLF15) is a key regulator of podocyte differentiation. The Journal of Biological Chemistry. 2012;**287**(23):19122-19135. DOI: 10.1074/jbc.M112.345983. Epub 2012 Apr 9

[107] Yu S, Yu L. Dexamethasone resisted Podocyte injury via stabilizing TRPC6 expression and distribution. Evidence-based Complementary and Alternative Medicine. 2012;**2012**:652059. DOI: 10.1155/2012/652059. Epub 2012 Apr 1

[108] Shimada M, Ishimoto T, Lee PY, Lanaspa MA, Rivard CJ, Roncal-Jimenez CA, et al. Toll-like receptor 3 ligands induce CD80 expression in human podocytes via an NF-κB-dependent pathway. Nephrology, Dialysis, Transplantation. 2012;**27**(1):81-89. DOI: 10.1093/ndt/gfr271. Epub 2011 May 26

[109] Lewko B, Waszkiewicz A, Maryn A, Gołos M, Latawiec E, Daca A, et al. Dexamethasone-dependent modulation of cyclic GMP synthesis in podocytes. Molecular and Cellular Biochemistry. 2015;**409**(1-2):243-253. DOI: 10.1007/s11010-015-2528-6. Epub 2015 Aug 14

[110] Ye M, Zheng J, Chen X, Chen X, Wu X, Lin X, et al. Prednisone inhibits the focal adhesion kinase/receptor activator of NF-κB ligand/mitogen-activated protein kinase signaling pathway in rats with adriamycin-induced nephropathy. Molecular Medicine Reports. 2015;**12**(5):7471-7478. DOI: 10.3892/mmr.2015.4370. Epub 2015 Sep 25

[111] Goode NP, Shires M, Khan TN, Mooney AF. Expression of

alpha-actinin-4 in acquired human nephrotic syndrome: A quantitative immunoelectron microscopy study. Nephrology, Dialysis, Transplantation. 2004;**19**(4):844-851. DOI: 10.1093/ndt/gfg620

[112] Zhao X, Khurana S, Charkraborty S, Tian Y, Sedor JR, Bruggman LA, et al. α actinin 4 (ACTN4) regulates glucocorticoid receptor-mediated transactivation and transrepression in podocytes. The Journal of Biological Chemistry. 2017;**292**(5):1637-1647. DOI: 10.1074/jbc.M116.755546. Epub 2016 Dec 20

[113] Anderberg RJ, Meek RL, Hudkins KL, Cooney SK, Alpers CE, Leboeuf RC, et al. Serum amyloid A and inflammation in diabetic kidney disease and podocytes. Laboratory Investigation. 2015;**95**:697

[114] Huang Y, Border WA, Yu L, Zhang J, Lawrence DA, Noble NA. A PAI-1 mutant, PAI-1R, slows progression of diabetic nephropathy. Journal of the American Society of Nephrology : JASN. 2008;**19**(2):329-338. DOI: 10.1681/ASN.2007040510. Epub 2008 Jan 23

[115] Wu J, Zheng C, Fan Y, Zeng C, Chen Z, Qin W, et al. Downregulation of microRNA-30 facilitates podocyte injury and is prevented by glucocorticoids. Journal of the American Society of Nephrology : JASN. 2014;**25**(1):92-104. DOI: 10.1681/ASN.2012111101. Epub 2013 Sep 12

[116] Jiang L, Hindmarch CC, Rogers M, Campbell C, Waterfall C, Coghill J, et al. RNA sequencing analysis of human podocytes reveals glucocorticoid regulated gene networks targeting non-immune pathways. Scientific Reports. 2016;**6**:35671. DOI: 10.1038/srep35671

[117] Querfeld U, Weber LT. Mycophenolate mofetil for sustained remission in nephrotic syndrome. Pediatric Nephrology. 2018;**33**(12):2253-2265. DOI: 10.1007/s00467-018-3970-y. Epub 2018 May 11

[118] Abo Zed SED, Hackl A, Bohl K, Ebert L, Kieckhöfer E, Müller C, et al. Mycophenolic acid directly protects podocytes by preserving the actin cytoskeleton and increasing cell survival. Scientific Reports. 15 Mar 2023;**13**(1):4281. DOI: 10.1038/s41598-023-31326-z. PMID: 36922538; PMCID: PMC10017704

[119] Lv W, Lou J, Zhang Y, Lian P, Qi D, Wang J. Mycophenolate mofetil inhibits hypertrophy and apoptosis of podocyte in vivo and in vitro. International Journal of Clinical and Experimental Medicine. 2015;**8**(10):19781-19790

[120] Romero F, Rodríguez-Iturbe B, Parra G, González L, Herrera-Acosta J, Tapia E. Mycophenolate mofetil prevents the progressive renal failure induced by 5/6 renal ablation in rats. Kidney International. 1999;**55**(3):945-955. DOI: 10.1046/j.1523-1755.1999.055003945.x

[121] Gipson DS, Trachtman H, Kaskel FJ, Greene TH, Radeva MK, Gassman JJ, et al. Clinical trial of focal segmental glomerulosclerosis in children and young adults. Kidney International. 2011;**80**(8):868-878. DOI: 10.1038/ki.2011.195. Epub 2011 Jul 6

[122] Cattran DC, Wang MM, Appel G, Matalon A, Briggs W. Mycophenolate mofetil in the treatment of focal segmental glomerulosclerosis. Clinical Nephrology. 2004;**62**(6):405-411. DOI: 10.5414/cnp62405

[123] Shen X, Zhang Y, Lin C, Weng C, Wang Y, Feng S, et al. Calcineurin inhibitors ameliorate PAN-induced podocyte injury through the NFAT-Angptl4 pathway. The Journal of Pathology. 2020;**252**(3):227-238. DOI: 10.1002/path.5512. Epub 2020 Sep 8

[124] Mallipattu SK, He JC. The podocyte as a direct target for treatment of glomerular disease? American Journal of Physiology. Renal Physiology. 2016;**311**(1):F46-F51. DOI: 10.1152/ajprenal.00184.2016. Epub 2016 Apr 20

[125] Li X, Zhang X, Li X, Wang X, Wang S, Ding J. Cyclosporine A protects podocytes via stabilization of cofilin-1 expression in the unphosphorylated state. Experimental Biology and Medicine (Maywood, N.J.). 2014;**239**(8):922-936. DOI: 10.1177/1535370214530365. Epub 2014 Apr 15

[126] Schlöndorff J, Del Camino D, Carrasquillo R, Lacey V, Pollak MR. TRPC6 mutations associated with focal segmental glomerulosclerosis cause constitutive activation of NFAT-dependent transcription. American Journal of Physiology. Cell Physiology. 2009;**296**(3):C558-C569. DOI: 10.1152/ajpcell.00077.2008. Epub 2009 Jan 7

[127] Wakamatsu A, Fukusumi Y, Hasegawa E, Tomita M, Watanabe T, Narita I, et al. Role of calcineurin (CN) in kidney glomerular podocyte: CN inhibitor ameliorated proteinuria by inhibiting the redistribution of CN at the slit diaphragm. Physiological Reports. 2016;**4**(6):e12679. DOI: 10.14814/phy2.12679

[128] Vollenbröker B, George B, Wolfgart M, Saleem MA, Pavenstädt H, Weide T. mTOR regulates expression of slit diaphragm proteins and cytoskeleton structure in podocytes. American Journal of Physiology. Renal Physiology. 2009;**296**(2):F418-F426. DOI: 10.1152/ajprenal.90319.2008. Epub 2008 Nov 19

[129] Allison SJ. Glomerular disease: mTOR in FSGS. Nature Reviews. Nephrology. 2017;**13**(5):260. DOI: 10.1038/nrneph.2017.42. Epub 2017 Mar 27

[130] Gödel M, Hartleben B, Herbach N, Liu S, Zschiedrich S, Lu S, et al. Role of mTOR in podocyte function and diabetic nephropathy in humans and mice. The Journal of Clinical Investigation. 2011;**121**(6):2197-2209. DOI: 10.1172/JCI44774. Epub 2011 May 23

[131] Zschiedrich S, Bork T, Liang W, Wanner N, Eulenbruch K, Munder S, et al. Targeting mTOR signaling can prevent the progression of FSGS. Journal of the American Society of Nephrology : JASN. 2017;**28**(7):2144-2157. DOI: 10.1681/ASN.2016050519. Epub 2017 Mar 7

[132] Fervenza FC, Fitzpatrick PM, Mertz J, Erickson SB, Liggett S, Popham S, et al. Mayo nephrology collaborative committee. Acute rapamycin nephrotoxicity in native kidneys of patients with chronic glomerulopathies. Nephrology, Dialysis, Transplantation. 2004;**19**(5):1288-1292. DOI: 10.1093/ndt/gfh079. Epub 2004 Feb 19

[133] Tumlin JA, Miller D, Near M, Selvaraj S, Hennigar R, Guasch A. A prospective, open-label trial of sirolimus in the treatment of focal segmental glomerulosclerosis. Clinical Journal of the American Society of Nephrology. 2006;**1**(1):109-116. DOI: 10.2215/CJN.00120605. Epub 2005 Nov 30

[134] Kershaw DB, Sedman AB, Kelsch RC, Bunchman TE. Recurrent focal segmental glomerulosclerosis in pediatric renal transplant recipients: Successful treatment with oral cyclophosphamide. Clinical Transplantation. 1994;**8**(6):546-549

[135] Cochat P, Kassir A, Colon S, Glastre C, Tourniaire B, Parchoux B, et al. Recurrent nephrotic syndrome after transplantation: Early treatment with plasmaphaeresis and cyclophosphamide. Pediatric Nephrology. 1993;7(1):50-54. DOI: 10.1007/BF00861567

[136] Dall'Amico R, Ghiggeri G, Carraro M, Artero M, Ghio L, Zamorani E, et al. Prediction and treatment of recurrent focal segmental glomerulosclerosis after renal transplantation in children. American Journal of Kidney Diseases. 1999;**34**(6):1048-1055. DOI: 10.1016/S0272-6386(99)70010-7

[137] Fornoni A, Sageshima J, Wei C, Merscher-Gomez S, Aguillon-Prada R, Jauregui AN, et al. Rituximab targets podocytes in recurrent focal segmental glomerulosclerosis. Science Translational Medicine. 2011;**3**(85):85ra46. DOI: 10.1126/scitranslmed.3002231

[138] Lanaret C, Anglicheau D, Audard V, Büchler M, Caillard S, Couzi L, et al. Rituximab for recurrence of primary focal segmental glomerulosclerosis after kidney transplantation: Results of a nationwide study. American Journal of Transplantation. 2021;**21**(9):3021-3033. DOI: 10.1111/ajt.16504. Epub 2021 Feb 23

[139] Canaud G, Zuber J, Sberro R, Royale V, Anglicheau D, Snanoudj R, et al. Intensive and prolonged treatment of focal and segmental glomerulosclerosis recurrence in adult kidney transplant recipients: A pilot study. American Journal of Transplantation. 2009;**9**(5):1081-1086. DOI: 10.1111/j.1600-6143.2009.02580.x. Epub 2009 Mar 16

[140] Lu Y, Lyons J, Tischer S, Woodside K, Park J. Efficacy and safety of a single-dose rituximab for prevention of focal segmental glomerulosclerosis recurrence after kidney transplant. American Journal of Transplantation. 2017;**17**(suppl 3)

[141] Auñón P, Polanco N, Pérez-Sáez MJ, Rodrigo E, Sancho A, Pascual J, et al. Pre-emptive rituximab in focal and segmental glomerulosclerosis patients at risk of recurrence after kidney transplantation. Clinical Kidney Journal. 2019;**14**(1):139-148. DOI: 10.1093/ckj/sfz120

[142] Hansrivijit P, Ghahramani N. Combined rituximab and plasmapheresis or plasma exchange for focal segmental glomerulosclerosis in adult kidney transplant recipients: A meta-analysis. International Urology and Nephrology. 2020;**52**(7):1377-1387. DOI: 10.1007/s11255-020-02462-6. Epub 2020 Apr 18

[143] Coady MJ, Wallendorff B, Lapointe JY. Characterization of the transport activity of SGLT2/MAP17, the renal low-affinity Na-glucose cotransporter. American Journal of Physiology. Renal Physiology [Internet]. 2017;**313**(2):F467-F474. DOI: 10.1152/ajprenal.00628.2016

[144] Kidney Disease: Improving Global Outcomes (KDIGO) CKD Work Group. KDIGO 2024 clinical practice guideline for the evaluation and management of chronic kidney disease. Kidney International [Internet]. 2024;**105**(4S):S117-S314. DOI: 10.1016/j.kint.2023.10.018

[145] Wheeler DC, Toto RD, Stefánsson BV, Jongs N, Chertow GM, Greene T, et al. A pre-specified analysis of the DAPA-CKD trial demonstrates the effects of dapagliflozin on major adverse kidney events in patients with IgA nephropathy. Kidney International [Internet]. 2021;**100**(1):215-224. DOI: 10.1016/j.kint.2021.03.033

[146] Anders HJ, Peired AJ, Romagnani P. SGLT2 inhibition requires reconsideration of fundamental paradigms in chronic kidney disease, "diabetic nephropathy", IgA nephropathy and podocytopathies with FSGS lesions. Nephrology, Dialysis, Transplantation [Internet]. 2022;**37**(9):1609-1615. DOI: 10.1093/ndt/gfaa329

[147] The EMPA-Kidney Collaborative Group, Herrington WG, Staplin N, Wanner C, Green JB, Hauske SJ, et al. Empagliflozin in patients with chronic kidney disease. The New England Journal of Medicine [Internet]. 2023;**388**(2):117-127. DOI: 10.1056/NEJMoa2204233

[148] Heerspink HJL, Stefánsson BV, Correa-Rotter R, Chertow GM, Greene T, Hou FF, et al. Dapagliflozin in patients with chronic kidney disease. The New England Journal of Medicine [Internet]. 2020;**383**(15):1436-1446. DOI: 10.1056/NEJMoa2024816

[149] Chan ATP, Tang SCW. Could SGLT2 inhibitors be the next "game changer" in focal segmental glomerulosclerosis? Nephrology, Dialysis, Transplantation [Internet]. 2022;**37**(9):1593-1594. DOI: 10.1093/ndt/gfac139

[150] Boeckhaus J, Gross O. Sodium-glucose cotransporter-2 inhibitors in patients with hereditary podocytopathies, Alport syndrome, and FSGS: A case series to better plan a large-scale study. Cells. 18 Jul 2021;**10**(7):1815. DOI: 10.3390/cells10071815

[151] Elkeraie A, Zyada R, Elrggal ME, Elrggal M. Safety of SGLT2 inhibitors in patients with different glomerular diseases treated with immunosuppressive therapies. European Journal of Clinical Pharmacology. 2023;**79**(7):961-966. DOI: 10.1007/s00228-023-03508-1

[152] Requião-Moura LR, Moscoso-Solorzano GT, Franco MF, Ozaki KS, Pacheco-Silva A, Kirsztajn GM, et al. Prognostic factors associated with poor graft outcomes in renal recipients with post-transplant glomerulonephritis. Clinical Transplantation. 2007;**21**(3):363-370

[153] Arai M, Wada A, Isaka Y, Akagi Y, Sugiura T, Miyazaki M, et al. In vivo transfection of genes for renin and angiotensinogen into the glomerular cells induced phenotypic change of the mesangial cells and glomerular sclerosis. Biochemical and Biophysical Research Communications. 1995;**206**(2):525-532

[154] Abuzeineh M, Aala A, Alasfar S, Alachkar N. Angiotensin II receptor 1 antibodies associate with post-transplant focal segmental glomerulosclerosis and proteinuria. BMC Nephrology. 2020;**21**(1):253

[155] Freiberger V, Amann K, Heemann U, Frank H. Effect of a triple blockade of the renin-angiotensin-system in recurrent focal segmental glomerulosclerosis after kidney transplantation. Transplant International. 2009;**22**(11):1110-1113

[156] Basu B, Angeletti A, Islam B, Ghiggeri GM. New and old anti-CD20 monoclonal antibodies for nephrotic syndrome. Where we are? Frontiers in Immunology. 2022;**13**:805697

[157] Ravani P, Colucci M, Bruschi M, Vivarelli M, Cioni M, DiDonato A, et al. Human or chimeric monoclonal anti-CD20 antibodies for children with nephrotic syndrome: A superiority randomized trial. Journal of the American Society of Nephrology : JASN. 2021;**32**(10):2652-2663

[158] Bernard J, Lalieve F, Sarlat J, Perrin J, Dehoux L, Boyer O, et al. Ofatumumab treatment for nephrotic syndrome recurrence after pediatric renal transplantation. Pediatric Nephrology. 2020;**35**(8):1499-1506

[159] Solomon S, Zolotnitskaya A, Del Rio M. Ofatumumab in post-transplantation recurrence of focal segmental glomerulosclerosis in a child. Pediatric Transplantation. 2019;**23**(4):e13413

[160] Reynolds BC, Lamb A, Jones CA, Yadav P, Tyerman KS, Geddes CC. UK experience of ofatumumab in recurrence of focal segmental glomerulosclerosis post-kidney transplant. Pediatric Nephrology. 2022;**37**(1):199-207

[161] Ural Z, Helvacı Ö, Özbaş B, Güz G, Derici Ü. Unexpected late response to ofatumumab in adult post-transplantation recurrent focal segmental glomerulosclerosis, case report. Transplantation Proceedings. 2022;**54**(6):1632-1635

[162] Delville M, Baye E, Durrbach A, et al. B7-1 blockade does not improve post–transplant nephrotic syndrome caused by recurrent FSGS. Journal of the American Society of Nephrology : JASN. 2016;**27**(8):2520-2527

[163] Shah Y, Almeshari K, Aleid H, et al. Successful treatment with abatacept in recurrent focal segmental glomerulosclerosis after kidney transplant. Experimental and Clinical Transplantation. 2019;**17**(Suppl. 1):178-180

[164] Alhasan KA, Alherbish A, Osman A, et al. Successful treatment of recurrent focal segmental glomerulosclerosis after transplantation in children: A single-center experience. Transplantation Proceedings. 2019;**51**(2):517-521

[165] Mühlbacher T, Amann K, Mahling M, et al. Successful long-term management of recurrent focal segmental glomerulosclerosis after kidney transplantation with costimulation blockade. Clinical Kidney Journal. 2021;**14**(6):1691-1693

[166] Grellier J, Del Bello A, Milongo D, Guilbeau-Frugier C, Rostaing L, Kamar N. Belatacept in recurrent focal segmental glomerulosclerosis after kidney transplantation. Transplant International. 2015;**28**(9):1109-1110

[167] Bitzan M, Babayeva S, Vasudevan A, Goodyer P, Torban E. TNFα pathway blockade ameliorates toxic effects of FSGS plasma on podocyte cytoskeleton and β3 integrin activation. Pediatric Nephrology. 2012;**27**(12):2217-2226

[168] Leroy S, Guigonis V, Bruckner D, Emal-Aglae V, Deschenes G, Bensman A, et al. Successful anti-TNFalpha treatment in a child with posttransplant recurrent focal segmental glomerulosclerosis. American Journal of Transplantation. 2009;**9**(4):858-861

[169] Hu QD, Tan RZ, Zou YX, Li JC, Fan JM, Kantawong F, et al. Synergism of calycosin and bone marrow-derived mesenchymal stem cells to combat podocyte apoptosis to alleviate adriamycin-induced focal segmental glomerulosclerosis. World Journal of Stem Cells. 2023;**15**(6):617-631

[170] Belingheri M, Lazzari L, Parazzi V, Groppali E, Biagi E, Gaipa G, et al. Allogeneic mesenchymal stem cell infusion for the stabilization of focal segmental glomerulosclerosis. Biologicals. 2013;**41**(6):439-445

[171] Suthar K, Vanikar AV, Trivedi HL. Renal transplantation in primary focal segmental glomerulosclerosis using a tolerance induction protocol. Transplantation Proceedings. 2008;**40**(4):1108-1110

[172] Allard L, Kwon T, et al. Treatment by immunoadsorption for recurrent focal segmental glomerulosclerosis after paediatric kidney transplantation: A multicentre French cohort. Nephrology, Dialysis, Transplantation. 2018;**33**:954-963

[173] Rainaa R, Wang J, et al. Extracorporeal therapies in the treatment

of focal segmental glomerulosclerosis. Blood Purification. 2020;**49**:513-523

[174] Padmanabhan A, Connelly-Smith L, et al. Guidelines on the use of therapeutic apheresis in clinical practice – Evidence-based approach from the writing Committee of the American Society for apheresis: The eighth special issue. Journal of Clinical Apheresis. 2019;**34**:171-354

[175] Tavera M. Chapter artificial liver support systems. Artificial Liver Support Systems. DOI: 10.5772/intechopen.109843

[176] Sharma M, Sharma R, McCarthy ET, Savin VJ. The focal segmental glomerulosclerosis permeability factor: Biochemical characteristics and biological effects. Experimental Biology and Medicine. 2004;**229**:85-98

[177] Vlachopanos G, Georgalis A, Gakiopoulou H. Plasma exchange for the recurrence of primary focal segmental glomerulosclerosis in adult renal transplant recipients: A meta-analysis. Journal of Transplantation. 2015;**2015**:639628. DOI: 10.1155/2015/639628. Epub 2015 Nov 30

[178] Dantal J, Godfrin Y, Koll R, et al. Antihuman immunoglobulin affinity immunoadsorption strongly decreases proteinuria in patients with relapsing nephrotic syndrome. Journal of the American Society of Nephrology : JASN. 1998;**9**:1709-1015

[179] Naciri Bennania H, Bonzi JY, Noble J, Terrec F, Motte L, Imerzoukene F, et al. Immunoadsorption for recurrent primary focal segmental glomerulosclerosis on kidney allografts: A single-center experience and literature review. Blood Purification. 2020;**49**(3):322-333. DOI: 10.1159/000504244

[180] Okwuonu CG et al. Therapeutic apheresis in kidney transplantation: Emerging trends. Journal of Clinical Apheresis. 2024;**39**:e22119

[181] Bible E. Immunoadsorption combined with membrane filtration might enhance desensitization. Nature Reviews Nephrology. 2014;**10**:125. DOI: 10.1038/nrneph.2014.5

[182] Lionaki S, Vlachopanos G, Georgalis A, et al. Individualized scheme of immunoadsorption for the recurrence of idiopathic focal segmental glomerulosclerosis in the graft: A single center experience. Renal Failure. 2015;**37**(5):777-783

[183] Muso E, Mune M, Hirano T, Hattori M, Kimura K, Watanabe T, et al. Immediate therapeutic efficacy of low-density lipoprotein apheresis for drug-resistant nephrotic syndrome: Evidence from the short-term results from the POLARIS study. Clinical and Experimental Nephrology. Jul 2015;**19**(3):379-386. DOI: 10.1007/s10157-014-0996-8

[184] Raina R, Krishnappa V, Sanchez-Kazi C, Quiroga A, Twombley KE, Mathias R, et al. Dextran-sulfate plasma adsorption lipoprotein apheresis in drug resistant primary focal segmental glomerulosclerosis patients: Results from a prospective, multicenter, single-arm intervention study. Frontiers in Pediatrics. 3 Dec 2019;**7**:454. DOI: 10.3389/fped.2019.00454

[185] Shah L, Hooper DK, Okamura D, Wallace D, Moodalbail D, Gluck C, et al. LDL-apheresis-induced remission of focal segmental glomerulosclerosis recurrence in pediatric renal transplant recipients. Pediatric Nephrology. Nov 2019;**34**(11):2343-2350. DOI: 10.1007/s00467-019-04296-6

Chapter 3

Overcoming the Hurdle: HLA Mismatch and Desensitization Therapy in Kidney Transplantation

Karen Courville and Norman Bustamante

Abstract

The success of kidney transplantation hinges on compatibility between donor and recipient. However, a major obstacle lies in the presence of Human Leukocyte Antigen (HLA) mismatches. These protein markers on cell surfaces trigger the recipient's immune system to attack the transplanted kidney. This challenge is particularly prevalent in patients who have developed antibodies against mismatched HLA antigens due to prior transplants, blood transfusions, or pregnancies. This chapter delves into the complexities of HLA mismatch and its impact on kidney transplant outcomes. We explore the immunological basis for rejection and discuss the limitations of traditional matching strategies. Desensitization therapy emerges as a beacon of hope, offering a range of techniques to reduce pre-existing anti-HLA antibodies and improve transplant success rates. We deepen into the mechanisms of desensitization, exploring various approaches like plasma exchange, immunoadsorption, and B-cell depletion therapies; we mention the most common side effects of these treatments; and the chapter concludes by examining the current state of desensitization protocols and their potential to revolutionize kidney transplantation for a broader range of patients.

Keywords: HLA antibodies, DSA, desensitization, kidney transplant, T-cells, B-cells, antibody

1. Introduction

HLA matching is crucial for successful kidney transplantation, promoting engraftment and reducing complications. HLAs are proteins found on the surface of cells; they are essential for the immune system's recognition of self and nonself and in kidney transplantation, HLAs determine compatibility between the donor and recipient. These genes are highly polymorphic, meaning they have many different variants [1].

The HLA genes are encoded on chromosome 6 and are inherited in Mendelian fashion, with one linked set of genes (haplotype) inherited intact from each parent and the system is divided into three classes: Class I HLAs, found on almost all nucleated cells in the body, are important for detecting infected or abnormal cells and present peptides from inside the cell to cytotoxic T cells. Class II HLAs are found primarily on antigen-presenting cells (APCs), such as dendritic cells, macrophages, and B cells. They present peptides from outside the cell to helper T cells and are crucial for immune responses against pathogens. Class III HLAs encode various immune-related proteins, including components of the complement system, but are not directly involved in antigen presentation [2, 3].

When there is an HLA mismatch in transplantation, the recipient's immune system recognizes the transplanted organ as foreign due to differences in HLA proteins. A cell-mediated immune response occurs *via* cytotoxic T cells (CD8+ T cells), that recognize the HLA disparities and attack the transplanted tissue, leading to rejection. The severity of rejection depends on the degree of HLA mismatch. Also, an antibody-mediated immune response can occur, and B cells produce antibodies against the foreign HLA antigens. These antibodies can cause acute or chronic rejection. The chronic rejection may lead to graft dysfunction over time [4, 5].

To prevent rejection, transplant recipients receive immunosuppressive medications. Pretransplant, HLA typing assesses compatibility between donor and recipient, because better HLA matches, improve transplant success. There are highly sensitized kidney transplant patients who have developed antibodies that can pose challenges during transplantation, secondary to previous blood transfusions, pregnancy in women, and previous kidney transplants [6, 7]. These 30% of patients, highly sensitized, often face prolonged waiting times for a compatible kidney. Desensitization protocols are strategies used to reduce pre-existing antibodies in highly sensitized kidney transplant recipients that have high levels of donor-specific antibodies (DSAs), making it challenging to find a compatible donor [8, 9].

2. Mechanisms of desensitization

Desensitization is a process in which immunomodulating therapies are administered to transplant candidates as a means to eliminate or reduce HLA antibody levels in order to enable transplantation and avoid the development of antibody-mediated rejection [10].

HLA desensitization can be performed on both deceased and living donors. The objective of desensitization is the same in both scenarios, however, due to the unpredictable time of performing the deceased donor transplant, the protocols used are different. There is no uniformly accepted desensitization protocol, but there are three mechanisms: removal of antibodies, inhibition of antibody production, or use of immunoglobulins [11].

2.1 Removal of antibodies

Antibodies removal can be done by plasma exchange plasmapheresis (PP) or immunoadsorption (IA).

There are two main techniques used for plasmapheresis: centrifuge-based and membrane-based. Centrifuge-based plasmapheresis uses a centrifuge spinning the blood at high speeds to separate its components [12]. This technique is often preferred for its ability to handle larger blood volumes and for procedures requiring the collection of specific blood components, like platelets, alongside plasma removal [13]. However, it can be less mobile and requires a more complex setup compared to the other method. Membrane-based plasmapheresis is a technique that utilizes a different type of machine. Here, blood is passed through a special filter with tiny pores. The pores are large enough to allow plasma to pass through but small enough to retain blood cells. Plasma containing the unwanted antibodies gets separated from the blood cells on one side of the membrane. The blood cells (red blood cells, white blood cells, and platelets) remain on the other side of the membrane and are recirculated back into the recipient's bloodstream. The unwanted antibodies get discarded in the separated plasma [14].

This technique offers advantages like being more portable and potentially gentler on blood cells. However, it may not be suitable for procedures requiring the collection of other blood components or for processing very large blood volumes and it removes various proteins from the plasma, including some that might not be harmful [15].

Plasmapheresis removes immunoglobulins (Ig) in a nonspecific manner, resulting in a decrease in plasma proteins, coagulation factors, circulating antibodies, and immune complexes. It is necessary to replace the plasma removed. The solution used to replace plasma in plasmapheresis depends on several factors, including the patient's condition and the specific goals of the treatment, and it can be albumin, fresh frozen plasma, or a combination of albumin and saline solution. Albumin is a common choice because it is readily available and has minimal risk of causing allergic reactions, though is expensive [16]. Fresh Frozen Plasma (FFP) is plasma collected from healthy donors and frozen to preserve its components, and it is used when the patient also needs to replace clotting factors or other proteins present in plasma. There is a slightly higher risk of allergic reactions compared to albumin. The combination of albumin and saline is a saline solution (salt water) mixed with albumin that helps maintain blood volume, while albumin provides some protein function. This combination can be a good option when both volume replacement and some protein replacements are needed, but the risk of allergic reactions to FFP needs to be avoided [17].

Immunoadsorption (IA) has a high affinity for IgG and consequently decreases IgG type autoantibodies. This is a selective alternative for the selective removal of IgG antibodies, without effect on other plasma proteins including coagulation factors. The procedure utilizes columns packed with special beads that have a high affinity for specific molecules, particularly antibodies [18]. These beads are designed to target certain types of human leukocyte antigens (HLAs), which are proteins on cell surfaces that can trigger immune rejection. Most of the IA columns used are staphylococcal protein A columns (sepharose-bound staphylococcal protein A columns), which binds to IgG1, IgG2, and IgG4 antibodies, however, it has little affinity to IgG3 antibodies. The recipient's blood is passed through these columns. As the blood flows, the targeted antibodies get hooked onto the beads by their specific binding properties, and the blood, now depleted of the unwanted antibodies, is then returned to the recipient's circulation [19].

The advantage of immunoadsorption over plasmapheresis is the greater affinity for IgG with greater removal of antibodies and elimination of replacing volume with fresh plasma, but with a disadvantage, since the presence of anti-HLA IgG3 antibodies has been suggested in patients who develop acute and chronic antibody-mediated rejection. Besides, since immunoadsorption only removes the targeted antibodies, there is reduced blood loss, which can be beneficial for patients who might already have low blood volume [20].

2.2 Inhibition of antibody production

There are some steps before an antibody is produced. As previously mentioned, an APC attaches to the antigen, breaking it down into smaller pieces that are attached to the major histocompatibility-II complex (MHC-II). A T-cell, a helper T-cell, will bind to this MHC-II, and this activation also initiates B-cells. This activated B-cell will become a plasma cell, with the capacity to produce antibodies, or a memory cell, capable of remembering antigens for future production of antibodies. An antibody is produced to act upon a specific antigen, and plasma cells can produce millions of antibodies in a few days to protect the body [21].

In a desensitization protocol before a kidney transplant, inhibition of antibodies refers to suppressing the production or activity of antibodies that could attack the donor's kidney. This is crucial because these antibodies, specifically donor-specific antibodies (DSAs), can trigger rejection after the transplant [22].

There are some specific proteins on the surface of B cells. There is a protein called CD20, and is expressed on multiple populations of mature and immature B cells, as a transmembrane non-glycosylated phosphoprotein. Rituximab is a murine monoclonal antibody directed against the CD20 molecule, and when infused, it binds specifically to the CD20 protein on the B cell surface [23].

Rituximab recruits' components of the recipient's immune system, particularly macrophages. These macrophages engulf and destroy the B cells coated with rituximab, depleting populations of B cells that express CD20 *via* complement cytotoxicity, causing a decrement of the number of B cells present in the peripheral blood circulation within one to three days of the administration, and complete B cell depletion in most of the patients within one to six weeks [24].

With fewer B cells, the production of harmful DSAs is significantly reduced. This helps create a more favorable environment for the transplanted kidney. Rituximab might also have a broader effect on the immune system, potentially dampening the overall immune response and reducing the risk of rejection.

Rituximab does not eliminate B cells permanently; they eventually regenerate, and antibody production can resume in a period over 6–12 months after completing treatment because the CD20 molecule is not found on precursor B cells or mature plasma cells [25].

Rituximab is typically used alongside other desensitization methods like plasmapheresis or immunoadsorption. The specific timing of administration can vary depending on the desensitization protocol.

2.3 Immunoglobulins

Immunoglobulins, also widely known as antibodies, are Y-shaped proteins produced by plasma cells (a type of white blood cell) in the immune system. They play a critical role in defense against pathogens, like bacteria, viruses, and toxins. Each immunoglobulin is unique and designed to recognize and bind to a specific antigen, a foreign molecule on the surface of a pathogen. There are five types of immunoglobulins: IgG, IgA, IgM, IgE, and IgD. IgG is the most common type, accounting for about 80% of circulating antibodies. IgA is abundant in mucous membranes, like lungs and intestines. IgM is produced in response to a new infection and helps activate the immune system. IgE is involved in allergic reactions and IgD is still under investigation, but it is believed to play a role in B cell activation [26].

Once an immunoglobulin binds to its specific antigen, it can trigger various immune responses to neutralize the threat, such as preventing pathogens from attaching to healthy cells, agglutination of pathogens, and complement activation.

Immunoglobulins can also be produced in a lab and used as therapeutic agents. For example, intravenous immunoglobulin (IVIG) therapy contains a mixture of antibodies from healthy donors and it is used to treat people with immune deficiencies or certain autoimmune diseases [27].

In kidney transplantation, IVIG also has a wide range of applications, such as desensitization therapy, treatment of antibody-mediated rejection (AMR), application in ABO-incompatible kidney transplantation (ABOi-KT), and treatment of various viral infections, including human parvovirus B19 (HPV-B19), polyoma BK virus, and cytomegalovirus (CMV) [27].

Intravenous immune globulin (IVIG) produces an immunomodulatory effect through inhibition of the generation of inflammatory cytokines, activation of complement, and inhibition of production of antibodies. When used in highly sensitized patients results in reduced allosensitization, by decreasing anti-HLA antibodies, which can lessen ischemia-reperfusion injuries and can contribute to successful long-term allograft outcomes for cardiac and renal allograft recipients [28].

In patients with high levels of preformed anti-HLA antibodies (high Panel Reactive Antibody [PRA]), transplant rates are extremely low because they remain wait list for longer times. A randomized controlled trial (RCT) on desensitizing patients awaiting kidney transplantation with a 2 year follow-up period after kidney transplant, found that intravenous immunoglobulin (IVIg) was better than placebo in reducing allosensitization in those highly sensitized patients and that transplant rates were improved with IVIg therapy [29].

3. Desensitization protocols

Desensitization protocols in kidney transplant patients are constantly evolving. No single standardized protocol exists and the approach is tailored to each patient based on factors like severity of sensitization (i.e., the level and type of antibodies present) and donor availability (or finding a compatible donor despite the antibodies). The goal is to reduce or eliminate pre-existing antibodies that could attack a transplanted kidney [30]. In a general way, there is an assessment of the severity of sensitization and the patient's overall health and there is an evaluation of a suitable approach for this patient. HLA desensitization strategies are diverse and vary at each transplant center depending on clinical experience and preference because there is no conclusive evidence favoring one technique over another [31].

3.1 Plasmapheresis with low dose IVIG

This protocol was used in HLA-incompatible living donor kidney transplantation. Patients underwent plasmapheresis (PP) every other day and low-dose cytomegalovirus hyperimmune globulin (CMV-Ig) 100 mg/kg after each plasmapheresis. Additionally, the protocol included initiating tacrolimus (trough target level of 8–12 ng/mL) and mycophenolate mofetil (2 g/d) 2–3 weeks before transplant. Patients with low DSA titers (<1/8) receive 2–3 sessions, while those with DSA antibodies in titers >1/128 receive 6–10 sessions [8, 32].

The transplant is performed if the cross-match test is negative. Induction is performed with daclizumab. Plasmapheresis is continued for 2–5 sessions after transplantation depending on DSA titers. This scheme showed significantly better long-term patient survival compared to the group of highly sensitized patients (PRA > 80%) who remained on dialysis or the dialysis group, but on the transplant waiting list [33, 34].

The protocol has been modified using induction with anti-thymocyte antibodies or basiliximab (since 2004), and additional use of rituximab or splenectomy; however, 39-43% of patients presented AMR. Patient and graft survival was 86 and 78% respectively at 15 months [35, 36].

The disadvantage of this scheme is the high costs of the therapy, which may involve several sessions of plasmapheresis to reduce the values of DSA antibodies pretransplant, and posttransplant plasmapheresis to prevent increases in DSA antibodies and acute rejection humoral [37].

3.2 High-dose IVIG

The advantage of this high dose of immunoglobulins (IVIG) (2 g/kg) without plasmapheresis (PP) protocol, is that it can be applied to deceased donor transplants. IVIg dose 2 g/kg monthly for 4 months with additional doses at 12 and 24 months if the patient has not received a kidney transplant. This regimen induces a 10% decrease in PRA levels compared to placebo and persists for 6 weeks after the last dose of IVIG. No difference was observed in transplant rate at 1 year, however, at 2 years 35% of patients with high-dose IVIG were transplanted. The incidence of acute rejection in the IVIG group was high (53%) compared to placebo (10%) [28].

The high-dose IVIG protocol has been modified with 2 g/Kg administered on days 0 and 30, adding rituximab 1 g on days 7 and 22, achieving a decrease in PRA from 77 to 44%. Patient and graft survival was 100 and 94% respectively at 12 months. Fifty percent of patients presented acute rejection and 30% presented antibody-mediated rejection (ABMR) [38].

Among the different desensitization protocols used, high-dose IVIG (2–3 g/Kg) (group 1) vs. PP/low-dose IVIG + rituximab 375 mg/m^2 single dose pretransplant (group 2) vs. PP/low dose IVIG + rituximab 375 m/m2 + pretransplant anti-thymocyte globulin (group 3) with monitoring of DSA levels post-renal transplant, it is concluded that PP-based regimens showed greater success in negating the results of positive cross-matching (group 1 = 38%, group 2 = 84%, group 3 = 88%). In transplant patients, humoral rejection (AMR) was 80% in the high-dose IVIG group compared to 37 and 29% in the PP groups [39].

4. Complications of anti-HLA desensitization therapy

Desensitization is a complex process with potential side effects associated with the medications used. There are some key points to take knowledge and explain to patients before going through the process.

4.1 Rejection

Desensitization protocols have shown a 2-year survival of the patient and the graft of 95 and 86% respectively, however, with a high percentage of acute cellular rejection (36%) and acute humoral rejection (28%), significantly higher than non-sensitized patients (10%), regardless of the desensitization protocol used and the type of induction used (daclizumab, anti-thymocyte globulin, or alentuzumab). Five-year follow-up has shown 69% graft survival in desensitized patients, significantly lower than in non-sensitized patients (81%) [40].

An increased risk of antibody-mediated rejection and the development of transplant glomerulopathy has been observed, which is a type of lesion unique to renal transplantation, characterized in renal biopsy by thickening of the glomerular capillary and double contour formation. This glomerulopathy can occur in up to 30% of desensitized patients who have developed acute humoral rejection, reducing kidney graft survival to 35% at 28 months [39].

4.2 Infections

Immunosuppressive medications used along with desensitization can weaken the immune system, making the patient more susceptible to infections. There is a reduced ability to fight new infections due to difficulty recognizing and eliminating new pathogens encountered after transplantation. Also, reactivation of latent infections can occur, as viruses or bacteria can remain in a dormant state. Immunosuppression can reactivate these latent infections, leading to serious illness, like CMV.

Using the data extrapolated from findings in ABO-incompatible transplants, due to the similarity of desensitization protocols used, studies have not shown an increased risk of infections compared to transplant patients without desensitization [41].

There are various strategies, used for avoiding infections in these patients, such as the use of prophylactic medication, ensuring up-to-date vaccinations before and after transplantation, and regularly monitoring patients for signs of infection and treating them promptly [42].

4.3 Malignancy

Immunosuppressant medications used in desensitization, particularly those that target B cells and T cells, can weaken the immune system's ability to fight abnormal cells that could develop into cancer.

Certain medications might have a more significant impact on the immune system compared to others, and underlying health conditions, age, and lifestyle habits can also influence cancer risk. Some studies have shown a possible association between desensitization and a slightly higher risk of certain malignancies, particularly non-melanoma skin cancers. Studies to evaluate the risk of malignancy in HLA-incompatible patients are limited, so the findings are extrapolated from ABO-incompatible patients, and no increased risk of cancer has been found in this HLA-incompatible group [43–45].

4.4 Other

Plasmapheresis can lower blood pressure, and cause muscle cramps, fatigue, and dizziness. There is also a risk of infection at the catheter insertion site. Immunoadsorption can also cause low blood pressure, fatigue, and dizziness. Additionally, there is a slight risk of allergic reactions to the column materials used in the process.

The potential benefits of a successful kidney transplant, particularly for patients with limited options, often outweigh the theoretical increased risk of malignancy or infections associated with desensitization therapy [46].

5. New medications for HLA desensitization

There are new and emerging drugs being explored for desensitization therapy in kidney transplants beyond plasmapheresis and intravenous immunoglobulin (IVIG) (**Box 1**).

There are anti-CD38 monoclonal antibodies that target a protein called CD38 present on the surface of various immune cells, including plasma cells that produce antibodies. They work by depleting plasma cells, thereby decreasing antibody production. Examples include Daratumumab and Isatuximab [47].

B-cell modulators target specific pathways involved in B cell activation and antibody production, inhibiting various signaling molecules crucial for B cell function. Ibrutinib and atacicept are still under investigation in the context of desensitization therapy.

Complement Inhibitors work by blocking specific steps in the complement cascade, preventing the complement system from attacking the transplanted kidney. Eculizumab and Eculizumab/Ravulizumab combination therapy, are already used to treat antibody-mediated rejection (AMR) in some kidney transplant patients [48]. Their role in desensitization protocols before transplantation is still being explored, with ongoing research to identify the most effective timing and combinations with other therapies. Use of eculizumab in living donor kidney recipients with pretransplant DSAs but negative crossmatches were given eculizumab injections (at days 0 and 1, then weekly for 1 month, thereafter every 2 weeks) for 1-year posttransplant.

Researchers are actively exploring various drugs with the potential to modulate the immune response and promote tolerance toward the transplanted kidney. Some of these drugs are already used as part of standard immunosuppressive regimens after transplantation.

1. Removal of anti-HLA antibodies
   a. Plasmapheresis
   b. Immunoadsorption
   c. IdeS
2. Depletion of antibody-producing cells
   a. Naïve and memory B cells: rituximab (anti-CD20)
   b. Plasma cells: bortezomib (proteosomal inhibitor)
3. Inhibition of antibody and complement-system cascade
   a. IVIg
   b. Complement inhibitors
      i. Eculizumab (C5a inhibitor)
      ii. C1 inhibitor
4. Inhibition of cytokines and inflammation
   a. IVIg
   b. Tocilizumab (anti-IL-6 receptor blocker)
   c. Belatacept (co stimulation blocker)

IdeS, immunoglobulin G-degrading enzymeof Streptococcus pyogenes; IL-6, interleukin 6; IVIg, intravenous immuneglobulin.

Box 1.
Agents used in desensitization protocols of kidney transplant.

Belatacept (costimulation blockade agent), Carfilzomib (proteasome inhibitor), and Alemtuzumab have diverse mechanisms of action, but they generally aim to dampen the overall immune response and reduce the risk of rejection. Their role specifically in desensitization protocols is still under investigation, with a focus on optimizing their use alongside other desensitization techniques [49, 50].

Bortezomib inhibits proteasomes leads to apoptosis of B cells. It has been used together with PP and rituximab, showing a significant decrease in anti-HLA antibodies [51].

Interleukin-6 (IL-6) receptor antagonist (Tocilizumab) is a monoclonal antibody directed against the interleukin 6 receptor. It blocks the activity of interleukin 6 and may interfere with plasmablasts/plasma cells, thereby decreasing the production of DSAs. It has been used in a small number of patients who failed desensitization with IVIg, plasmapheresis, and rituximab [52].

IdeS (immunoglobulin G [IgG]-degrading enzyme of *Streptococcus pyogenes*) is an extracellular cysteine proteinase produced by *S. pyogenes* that specifically cleaves all four human subclasses of IgG at the lower hinge region, generating 1 F(abo)2 fragment and 1 Fc fragment, and thereby inhibiting both Fc-mediated phagocytosis and bacterial killing. Because this IgG cleaving effect abrogates antibody-dependent and complement-mediated responses [53].

6. Non-DSA antibodies

There is growing evidence that some anti-HLA antibodies might not significantly affect long-term graft outcomes. These are often referred to as "non-pathogenic" or "non-DSA" antibodies. These antibodies might target less critical HLA molecules or have weaker binding properties that do not trigger a strong immune response. They might not activate the complement system, reducing their potential to damage the kidney. Despite the presence of potentially non-influencing antibodies, some transplant centers might still prioritize strategies to reduce overall antibody levels before transplantation, especially if strong DSAs are also present. This approach aims to minimize the overall risk of rejection. The immune response can vary between patients, and an antibody that appears non-influencing in one case might have a negative impact in another [54, 55].

7. Conclusion

Desensitization therapy plays a vital role in expanding kidney transplant opportunities for patients who would otherwise face significant challenges due to high levels of antibodies against potential donor kidneys. These antibodies, particularly donor-specific antibodies (DSAs), can trigger rejection after transplantation.

Current desensitization protocols often combine procedures like plasmapheresis and immunoadsorption with medications like rituximab (anti-CD20) and intravenous immunoglobulin (IVIG) to reduce antibody production and dampen the immune response. However, research is actively exploring new and promising drugs for desensitization. These include anti-CD38 monoclonal antibodies, B-cell modulators, complement inhibitors, and novel immunomodulatory drugs.

While desensitization offers hope for more patients, it is crucial to understand that it is a complex process with potential complications. Careful monitoring and ongoing management are essential to ensure successful transplant outcomes. Consulting with a qualified transplant team is vital to determine if desensitization is the right approach and to explore the most suitable protocol based on individual needs and the latest advancements in this evolving field.

Author details

Karen Courville[1,2]* and Norman Bustamante[1]

1 Hospital Dr. Gustavo N. Collado, Chitré, Herrera, Panama

2 Instituto de Ciencias Médicas, Las Tablas, Los Santos, Panama

*Address all correspondence to: kavac7@gmail.com

References

[1] Alelign T, Ahmed MM, Bobosha K, Tadesse Y, Howe R, Petros B. Kidney transplantation: The challenge of human leukocyte antigen and its therapeutic strategies. Journal of Immunology Research. 2018;(1):5986740. Published 2018 Mar 5. DOI: 10.1155/2018/5986740

[2] Palvair J, Farhat I, Chaintreuil M, et al. The potential role of the leucocyte immunoglobulin-like receptors in kidney transplant rejection: A mini review. Transplant International. 2024;**37**:12995. DOI: 10.3389/ti.2024.12995

[3] Klein J, Sato A. The HLA system. First of two parts. The New England Journal of Medicine. 2000;**343**(10):702-709. DOI: 10.1056/NEJM200009073431006

[4] Rogers NM, Eng HS, Yu R, et al. Desensitization for renal transplantation: Depletion of donor-specific anti-HLA antibodies, preservation of memory antibodies, and clinical risks. Transplant International. 2011;**24**(1):21-29. DOI: 10.1111/j.1432-2277.2010.01138.x

[5] McKenna RM, Takemoto SK, Terasaki PI. Anti-HLA antibodies after solid organ transplantation. Transplantation. 2000;**69**(3):319-326. DOI: 10.1097/00007890-200002150-00001

[6] Molina J, Navas A, Aguera ML, Rodriguez-Benot A. Avances en la inmunología del trasplante renal. NefroPlus. 2018;**10**(2):11-19. Available from: https://www.revistanefrologia.com/es-avances-inmunologia-del-trasplante-renal-articulo-X1888970018633756

[7] Keith DS, Vranic GM. Approach to the highly sensitized kidney transplant candidate. Clinical Journal of the American Society of Nephrology. 2016;**11**(4):684-693. DOI: 10.2215/CJN.05930615

[8] Montgomery RA, Lonze BE, King KE, et al. Desensitization in HLA-incompatible kidney recipients and survival. The New England Journal of Medicine. 2011;**365**(4):318-326. DOI: 10.1056/NEJMoa1012376

[9] Valentin MO, Ruiz JC, Vega R, Martín C, Matesanz R, working group PATHI. Implementation of a national priority allocation system for hypersensitized patients in Spain, based on virtual crossmatch: Initial results. Transplantation Proceedings. 2016;**48**(9):2871-2875. DOI: 10.1016/j.transproceed.2016.09.024

[10] Marfo K, Lu A, Ling M, Akalin E. Desensitization protocols and their outcome. Clinical Journal of the American Society of Nephrology. 2011;**6**(4):922-936. DOI: 10.2215/CJN.08140910

[11] Tambur AR, Campbell P, Chong AS, et al. Sensitization in transplantation: Assessment of risk (STAR) 2019 working group meeting report. American Journal of Transplantation. 2020;**20**(10):2652-2668. DOI: 10.1111/ajt.15937

[12] Cervantes CE, Bloch EM, Sperati CJ. Therapeutic plasma exchange: Core curriculum 2023. American Journal of Kidney Diseases. 2023;**81**(4):475-492. DOI: 10.1053/j.ajkd.2022.10.017

[13] Sanoff SL, Balogun RA, Lobo PL. The role of therapeutic apheresis in high immunologic risk renal transplantation: A review of current trends. Seminars in Dialysis. 2012;**25**(2):193-200. DOI: 10.1111/j.1525-139X.2011.01032.x

[14] Mantilla J, Peña D, Molano-Triviño A, Zúñiga E, Castellanos-De La Hoz JC. Divide et Vinces, therapeutic apheresis in nephrological clinical practice. Blood Purification. 2024;**53**(3):162-169. DOI: 10.1159/000534455

[15] Kuppachi S, Axelrod DA. Desensitization strategies: Is it worth it? Transplant International. 2020;**33**(3):251-259. DOI: 10.1111/tri.13532

[16] Ridel C, Kissling S, Mesnard L, Hertig A, Rondeau É. Échanges plasmatiques en néphrologie : Techniques et indications [plasma exchange in nephrology: Indications and technique]. Néphrologie & Thérapeutique. 2017;**13**(1):43-55. DOI: 10.1016/j.nephro.2016.12.002

[17] McLeod BC. Plasma and plasma derivatives in therapeutic plasmapheresis. Transfusion. 2012;**52**(Suppl. 1):38S-44S. DOI: 10.1111/j.1537-2995.2012.03623.x

[18] Rostaing L, Congy N, Aarnink A, et al. Efficacy of immunoadsorption to reduce donor-specific alloantibodies in kidney-transplant candidates. Experimental and Clinical Transplantation. 2015;**13** (Suppl. 1):201-206

[19] Rostaing L, Maggioni S, Hecht C, et al. Efficacy and safety of tandem hemodialysis and immunoadsorption to desensitize kidney transplant candidates. Experimental and Clinical Transplantation. 2015;**13** (Suppl. 1):165-169

[20] Maillard N, Absi L, Claisse G, Masson I, Alamartine E, Mariat C. Protein A-based immunoadsorption is more efficient than conventional plasma exchange to remove circulating anti-HLA antibodies. Blood Purification. 2015;**40**(2):167-172. DOI: 10.1159/000437041

[21] Altulea D, van den Born JC, Diepstra A, et al. Memory B-cell derived donor-specific antibodies do not predict outcome in sensitized kidney transplant recipients: A retrospective single-center study. Frontiers in Immunology. 2024;**15**:1360627. DOI: 10.3389/fimmu.2024.1360627

[22] Li X, Zhao Y, Sun W, et al. Neutrophil depletion attenuates antibody-mediated rejection in a renal transplantation mouse model. Clinical and Experimental Immunology. 2024;**216**(2):211-219. DOI: 10.1093/cei/uxad128

[23] Sood P, Hariharan S. Anti-CD20 blocker rituximab in kidney transplantation. Transplantation. 2018;**102**(1):44-58. DOI: 10.1097/TP.0000000000001849

[24] Tanaka A, Ide K, Tanaka Y, Ohira M, Tahara H, Ohdan H. B cell depletion with anti-CD20 mAb exacerbates anti-donor $CD4^+$ T cell responses in highly sensitized transplant recipients. Scientific Reports. 2021;**11**(1):18180. DOI: 10.1038/s41598-021-97748-9

[25] Sethi S, Ammerman N, Vo A, Jordan SC. Approach to highly sensitized kidney transplant candidates and a positive crossmatch. Advances in Chronic Kidney Disease. 2021;**28**(6):587-595. DOI: 10.1053/j.ackd.2021.09.004

[26] Justiz Vaillant AA, Jamal Z, Patel P, et al. Immunoglobulin. [updated 2023 Aug 28]. In: StatPearls [Internet]. Treasure Island (FL): StatPearls Publishing; 2024. Available from: https://www.ncbi.nlm.nih.gov/books/NBK513460/

[27] Hou YB, Chang S, Chen S, Zhang WJ. Intravenous immunoglobulin in kidney transplantation: Mechanisms of action, clinical applications, adverse effects, and hyperimmune globulin. Clinical Immunology. 2023;**256**:109782. DOI: 10.1016/j.clim.2023.109782

[28] Jordan SC, Tyan D, Stablein D, et al. Evaluation of intravenous immunoglobulin as an agent to lower allosensitization and improve transplantation in highly sensitized adult patients with end-stage renal disease: Report of the NIH $IG0_2$ trial. Journal of the American of Society of Nephrology. 2004;**15**(12):3256-3262. DOI: 10.1097/01.ASN.0000145878.92906.9F

[29] Jordan S, Cunningham-Rundles C, McEwan R. Utility of intravenous immune globulin in kidney transplantation: Efficacy, safety, and cost implications. American Journal of Transplantation. 2003;**3**(6):653-664. DOI: 10.1034/j.1600-6143.2003.00121.x

[30] Jordan SC, Reinsmoen N, Lai CH, et al. Desensitizing the broadly human leukocyte antigen-sensitized patient awaiting deceased donor kidney transplantation. Transplantation Proceedings. 2012;**44**(1):60-61. DOI: 10.1016/j.transproceed.2011.12.028

[31] Furian L, Bestard O, Budde K, et al. European consensus on the management of sensitized kidney transplant recipients: A Delphi study. Transplant International. 2024;**37**:12475. DOI: 10.3389/ti.2024.12475

[32] Zachary AA, Montgomery RA, Leffell MS. Factors associated with and predictive of persistence of donor-specific antibody after treatment with plasmapheresis and intravenous immunoglobulin. Human Immunology. 2005;**66**(4):364-370. DOI: 10.1016/j.humimm.2005.01.032

[33] Zachary AA, Montgomery RA, Ratner LE, et al. Specific and durable elimination of antibody to donor HLA antigens in renal-transplant patients. Transplantation. 2003;**76**(10):1519-1525. DOI: 10.1097/01.TP.0000090868.88895.E0

[34] Montgomery RA, Zachary AA. Transplanting patients with a positive donor-specific crossmatch: A single center's perspective. Pediatric Transplantation. 2004;**8**(6):535-542. DOI: 10.1111/j.1399-3046.2004.00214.x

[35] Khan MT, Hamid RB, Sarfaraz S, Lal N, Ahmed J, Luxmi S. Successful desensitization and kidney transplantation in the presence of donor-specific anti-human leukocyte antigen antibodies in kidney transplant recipients. Saudi Journal of Kidney Diseases and Transplantation. 2020;**31**(6):1432-1438. DOI: 10.4103/1319-2442.308365

[36] Magee CC, Felgueiras J, Tinckam K, Malek S, Mah H, Tullius S. Renal transplantation in patients with positive lymphocytotoxicity crossmatches: One center's experience. Transplantation. 2008;**86**(1):96-103. DOI: 10.1097/TP.0b013e318176ae2c

[37] Haririan A, Nogueira J, Kukuruga D, et al. Positive cross-match living donor kidney transplantation: Longer-term outcomes. American Journal of Transplantation. 2009;**9**(3):536-542. DOI: 10.1111/j.1600-6143.2008.02524.x

[38] Vo AA, Lukovsky M, Toyoda M, et al. Rituximab and intravenous immune globulin for desensitization during renal transplantation. The New England Journal of Medicine. 2008;**359**(3):242-251. DOI: 10.1056/NEJMoa0707894

[39] Stegall MD, Gloor J, Winters JL, Moore SB, Degoey S. A comparison of plasmapheresis versus high-dose IVIG desensitization in renal allograft recipients with high levels of donor specific alloantibody. American Journal of Transplantation. 2006;**6**(2):346-351. DOI: 10.1111/j.1600-6143.2005.01178.x

[40] Vo AA, Sinha A, Haas M, et al. Factors predicting risk for antibody-mediated rejection and graft loss in highly human leukocyte antigen sensitized patients transplanted after desensitization. Transplantation. 2015;**99**(7):1423-1430. DOI: 10.1097/TP.0000000000000525

[41] Kahwaji J, Sinha A, Toyoda M, et al. Infectious complications in kidney-transplant recipients desensitized with rituximab and intravenous immunoglobulin. Clinical Journal of the American Society of Nephrology. 2011;**6**(12):2894-2900. DOI: 10.2215/CJN.03710411

[42] Habicht A, Bröker V, Blume C, et al. Increase of infectious complications in ABO-incompatible kidney transplant recipients—A single centre experience. Nephrology, Dialysis, Transplantation. 2011;**26**(12):4124-4131. DOI: 10.1093/ndt/gfr215

[43] Couzi L, Manook M, Perera R, et al. Difference in outcomes after antibody-mediated rejection between abo-incompatible and positive cross-match transplantations. Transplant International. 2015;**28**(10):1205-1215. DOI: 10.1111/tri.12621

[44] Revuelta I, Ferreira R, Canha C, Piselli P, Verdirosi D, Tubita V, et al. Pre-transplant desensitization protocol and cancer risk in kidney transplantation. American Journal of Transplantation. 2015;**15**(Suppl. 3):1. Available from: https://atcmeetingabstracts.com/abstract/pre-transplant-desensitization-protocol-and-cancer-risk-in-kidney-transplantation/

[45] Yang CY, Lee CY, Yeh CC, Tsai MK. Renal transplantation across the donor-specific antibody barrier: Graft outcome and cancer risk after desensitization therapy. Journal of the Formosan Medical Association. 2016;**115**(6):426-433. DOI: 10.1016/j.jfma.2015.11.006

[46] Agarwal S, Maheshwari A, Bajpai M. Large volume plasmapheresis using a single-use immunoadsorption column: A cost-effective approach for desensitization in ABO-incompatible liver transplant. Journal of Clinical Apheresis. 2023;**38**(5):548-554. DOI: 10.1002/jca.22058

[47] Vo A, Ammerman N, Jordan SC. New therapies for highly sensitized patients on the waiting list. Kidney360. 2024:1-62. DOI: 10.34067/KID.0000000000000509. PMID: 38995690. [Epub ahead of print]

[48] Favi E, Cresseri D, Perego M, et al. Sequential administration of anti-complement component C5 eculizumab and type-2 anti-CD20 obinutuzumab for the treatment of early antibody-mediated rejection after kidney transplantation: A proof of concept. Clinical Immunology. 2024;**264**:110240. DOI: 10.1016/j.clim.2024.110240

[49] Ezekian B, Schroder PM, Mulvihill MS, et al. Pretransplant desensitization with costimulation blockade and proteasome inhibitor reduces DSA and delays antibody-mediated rejection in highly sensitized nonhuman primate kidney transplant recipients. Journal of the American of Society of Nephrology. 2019;**30**(12):2399-2411. DOI: 10.1681/ASN.2019030304

[50] Ge S, Pao A, Vo A, et al. Immunologic parameters and viral infections in patients desensitized with intravenous immunoglobulin and rituximab. Transplant Immunology. 2011;**24**(3):142-148. DOI: 10.1016/j.trim.2010.11.006

[51] Diwan TS, Raghavaiah S, Burns JM, Kremers WK, Gloor JM, Stegall MD. The impact of proteasome inhibition on alloantibody-producing plasma cells in vivo. Transplantation. 2011;**91**(5):536-541. DOI: 10.1097/TP.0b013e3182081333

[52] Vo AA, Choi J, Kim I, et al. A phase I/II trial of the interleukin-6 receptor-specific humanized monoclonal (tocilizumab) + intravenous immunoglobulin in difficult to desensitize patients. Transplantation. 2015;**99**(11):2356-2363. DOI: 10.1097/TP.0000000000000741

[53] Frick IM, Happonen L, Wrighton S, Nordenfelt P, Björck L. IdeS, a secreted proteinase of *Streptococcus pyogenes*, is bound to a nuclease at the bacterial surface where it inactivates opsonizing IgG antibodies. The Journal of Biological Chemistry. 2023;**299**(11):105345. DOI: 10.1016/j.jbc.2023.105345

[54] Bhutani S, Harris S, Carr M, et al. Evaluating the clinical relevance of antibodies against non-human leukocyte antigen in kidney transplantation. Antibodies (Basel). 2024;**13**(2):44. DOI: 10.3390/antib13020044

[55] Olszowska-Zaremba N, Gozdowska J, Zagożdżon R. Clinical significance of low pre-transplant donor specific antibodies (DSA) in living donor kidney recipients with negative complement-dependent cytotoxicity crossmatches (CDCXM), and negative flow cytometry crossmatches (FLXM)—A single-center experience. Transplant Immunology. 2022;**74**:101672. DOI: 10.1016/j.trim.2022.101672

Chapter 4

Kidney Paired Donation

Mohammad Hassan Al-thnaibat

Abstract

Kidney paired donation (KPD) offers a crucial solution to the challenges of organ transplantation, particularly for patients with immunological incompatibilities. By allowing incompatible donor-recipient pairs to exchange donors with other pairs, KPD significantly expands the donor pool, enhancing the likelihood of successful transplants. Advanced algorithms and desensitization techniques further optimize matching and compatibility. The ethical challenges, including equitable access and donor autonomy, require robust guidelines and transparency. As KPD programs evolve, incorporating strategies like altruistic donations and international collaborations can further enhance transplant success, making kidney transplants more accessible and equitable globally.

Keywords: kidney paired donation (KPD), desensitization, blood group, incompatibility, gender disparity, highly sensitized patients, donor pool expansion, non-directed altruistic donors (NDAD), ABO incompatible, transplants, kidney transplant chains, cross-organ exchange, international kidney exchange programs

1. Introduction

Kidney transplantation is the optimal treatment for patients with end-stage renal disease (ESRD), offering significantly better outcomes compared to dialysis [1]. However, the field of kidney transplantation faces numerous challenges, particularly in the area of living kidney donation. One of the most pressing issues is the shortage of compatible donors, exacerbated by the increasing demand for transplants [2].

Living donors are preferable to deceased donors due to better survival rates and shorter wait times [3]. Still, the discrepancy in transplant accessibility between male and female patients further complicates the landscape [4]. Women, often more likely to donate than receive, face additional barriers to transplantation, leading to disparities in outcomes [5].

Highly sensitized patients (HSP) who have developed high antibodies against human leukocyte antigens (HLA) due to previous transplants, blood transfusions, or pregnancies present another significant challenge. These antibodies make it exceedingly difficult to find compatible donors, substantially reducing the likelihood of successful transplantation for these individuals [6, 7]. Compatibility issues, particularly immunological barriers, remain one of the significant obstacles in kidney transplantation [8]. Certain groups, such as blood group O recipients, face specific challenges in finding compatible donors [9]. Blood group O recipients can only receive kidneys from blood group O donors, which limits their options and increases their wait times.

Developing effective strategies for expanding the donor pool is crucial to addressing these challenges. This includes leveraging innovative approaches like kidney paired donation (KPD), which can provide viable solutions for patients with incompatible donors. KPD allows for the creation of donation chains and exchanges that can match incompatible pairs with other pairs in similar situations, ultimately increasing the number of transplants.

Furthermore, unconventional strategies, such as incorporating non-directed altruistic donors (NDAD), facilitating ABO incompatible (ABOi) transplants, and exploring cross-organ exchanges like liver-kidney swaps can significantly enhance donor availability. The potential for international kidney exchange programs also offers a promising avenue for expanding the donor pool.

Overcoming the challenges of living kidney donation requires a multifaceted approach that includes understanding the unique needs of difficult-to-match recipients, addressing compatibility issues, and implementing innovative strategies to expand the donor pool. By doing so, we can move closer to ensuring that every patient, regardless of their immunological or demographic barriers, has access to life-saving kidney transplants [10].

2. Strategies to overcome immunological barriers in living kidney transplantation

In the field of living kidney transplantation (LKT), overcoming immunological barriers is crucial for ensuring successful outcomes. Desensitization and kidney paired donation (KPD) are crucial strategies for addressing the challenge of transplanting patients with donor-specific antibodies (DSAs).

2.1 Desensitization

Desensitization is a critical process for transplant candidates with donor-specific antibodies (DSAs) [11] to mitigate the risk of antibody-mediated rejection (AMR) and expand their access to potential donors. Traditional desensitization protocols involve a combination of plasmapheresis (PLEX), intravenous immunoglobulin (IVIG), and immunosuppressive agents, such as rituximab, which targets B cells, and daratumumab, which depletes plasma cells. These treatments aim to reduce preformed antibodies, making it feasible to perform transplants that would otherwise be contraindicated due to positive crossmatches. Despite their effectiveness, these methods are resource-intensive, require meticulous monitoring, and carry significant risks, including a higher incidence of AMR and decreased long-term graft survival. Studies from 2000 to 2010 involving 725 patients reported a 95% patient survival and 86% graft survival at two years, although acute rejection rates were 36% [12].

The heterogeneity in patient responses to desensitization necessitates individualized approaches, considering patients' immunological profiles and the type of allo-sensitizing events, such as previous transplants or pregnancies. Emerging strategies [13] use novel therapeutics like bispecific antibodies (anti-BCMA-CD3) and co-stimulation blockade agents like Belatacept, requiring further validation. Integrating immune-modulatory therapies, such as IL-6 inhibitors like tocilizumab, shows promise in reducing inflammation and supporting desensitization. Combining these with existing therapies could enhance DSA reduction and prevent rebound post-transplant. Adaptive clinical trial designs and standardized endpoints, like cPRA titers, are essential for refining desensitization protocols, improving transplant success rates and patient outcomes.

2.2 Kidney paired donation

KPD is an innovative solution that matches incompatible donor-recipient pairs with other pairs in similar situations, effectively creating chains of compatible transplants. This method increases the donor pool and enables more patients to receive transplants without the need for extensive desensitization. While KPD is generally less expensive and associated with lower risks of rejection and infection compared to desensitization, it comes with logistical challenges. Coordinating multiple simultaneous transplantations and addressing last-moment cancelations can be complex and require meticulous planning.

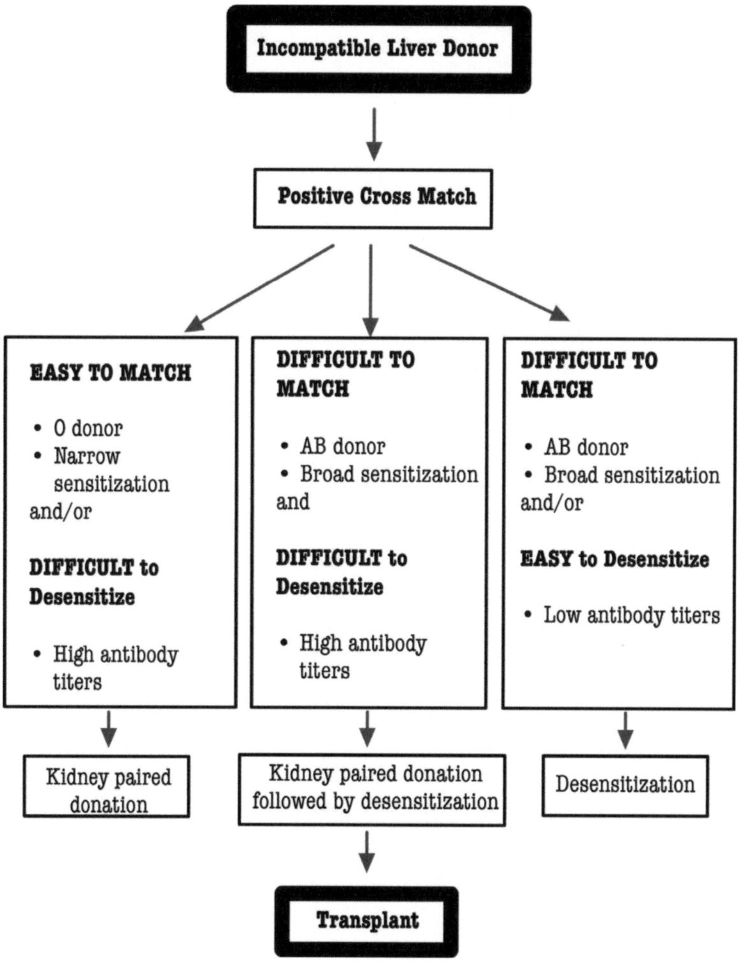

Figure 1.
Strategic approach for managing incompatible live donors based on matchability and antibody titers. It categorizes patients by ease of match and desensitization difficulty, guiding the choice between kidney paired donation (KPD), KPD with desensitization, or desensitization alone.

2.3 ABO incompatible versus paired donation

Both strategies have demonstrated significant success over the past decade, and emerging data supports their combined use. Comparing ABOitransplants to KPD, several factors stand out. ABOi transplants are generally less expensive and pose higher risk of rejection and infection due to advances in desensitization protocols. Long-term outcomes for ABOi transplants have also improved, making this a viable option for many patients. However, the logistical challenges inherent in KPD, such as the need for synchronized transplant surgeries and potential last-minute issues, make ABOi transplants an attractive alternative in certain scenarios. Desensitization and paired exchange are complementary strategies. Montgomery's proposed modality algorithm helps identify which donor/recipient phenotypes benefit from each approach. Patients who are easy to match but difficult to desensitize should opt for paired exchange, while those who are difficult to match but easy to desensitize should undergo desensitization. For those who are both difficult to match and desensitize, a combination of paired exchange and desensitization with an immunologically suited donor is recommended (**Figure 1**).

3. History of kidney paired donation

The concept of kidney paired donation (KPD) was first proposed by Felix Rapaport in 1986 [14]. He introduced the innovative idea of matching incompatible donor-recipient pairs with other such pairs to facilitate compatible transplants. This concept saw its first successful application in 1991 in South Korea, where the first KPD transplant was performed [15]. By 1999, the first paired exchange in Europe occurred at University Hospital in Basel, Switzerland. The United States conducted its first KPD transplant in 2000 [10], initially in New England and shortly after that by the Johns Hopkins team, further validating this approach and setting the stage for broader adoption.

Between 2000 and 2006 [16–19] KPD programs were established worldwide, creating multicenter and national registries. The Netherlands set a precedent in 2004 by successfully launching the first national KPD program globally, followed by establishing other national registries in many different countries. These registries have been instrumental in expanding the pool of potential matches, improving coordination, and increasing the success rates of KPD transplants. By the third quarter of 2010, over 1000 KPD transplants had been performed in the USA [10].

The academic and scientific community's recognition of the significance of KPD was solidified in 2012 when Alvin Roth was honored with the Nobel Prize in Economic Sciences for his contributions to the theory of stable allocations and market design [20], which included the development of matching algorithms used in KPD programs. In 2014 [21], the United States implemented advanced algorithms and software, significantly enhancing the efficiency of KPD matching processes. These technological advancements have transformed KPD into a more reliable and effective option for patients with incompatible donors, further validating its importance in the field.

As of 2024, improvements in KPD programs continue, focusing on refining matching algorithms, expanding donor pools, and increasing transplant accessibility and success rates. The evolution of KPD highlights the collaborative efforts of medical professionals, economists, and researchers to improve kidney transplantation outcomes for patients worldwide.

4. Modalities of kidney paired donation

The evolution of kidney paired donation (KPD) has introduced several innovative modalities to address donor-recipient incompatibilities. These advanced strategies improve match rates and transplant outcomes, particularly for highly sensitized patients and those with challenging blood types. Each modality offers unique advantages and faces specific challenges, enhancing the overall effectiveness and reach of KPD in providing life-saving transplants. By adopting these innovative approaches, KPD programs can significantly expand the donor pool and improve access to kidney transplantation for a broader range of patients.

4.1 Conventional KPD: closed loops and simultaneous transplants

A kidney transplant is deemed compatible if both the ABO blood group of the donor and recipient are matched and the crossmatch test is negative, which can be determined through either the Complement-Dependent Cytotoxicity (CDC) test or virtually (no donor-specific antibodies, DSA).

Conventional kidney-paired donation (KPD) involves direct exchanges between incompatible donor-recipient pairs, forming closed loops where transplants are conducted simultaneously. The simplest form is the two-way loop, where two incompatible pairs exchange kidneys such that each recipient receives a kidney from the donor of the other pair. This setup is straightforward and ensures both transplants occur simultaneously, minimizing the risk of donors backing out after their recipient has received a kidney. This is the simplest form of KPD, which requires pairs to have reciprocal or complementary incompatibilities (**Figure 2**).

As the number of participating pairs increases, the complexity of the exchanges can grow significantly. Entering more pairs into an exchange, such as 3-way or even up to 10-way loops, not only facilitates more transplants but also increases options for difficult-to-match patients, as complementary incompatibilities are not required. This

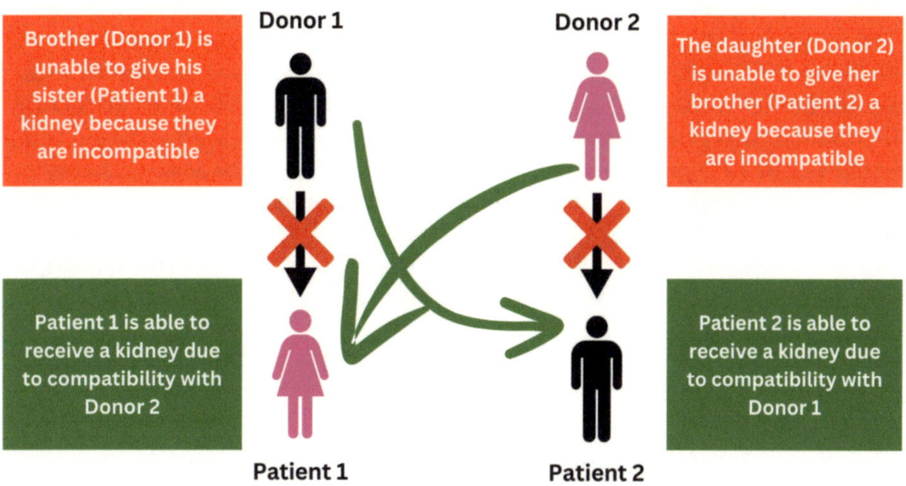

Figure 2.
This diagram illustrates a scenario in kidney paired donation where two incompatible donor-recipient pairs swap donors to facilitate transplants. In this example, Brother (Donor 1) and Daughter (Donor 2) are unable to donate directly to their respective siblings, Patient 1 and Patient 2, due to incompatibility. However, by swapping, Donor 1 donates to Patient 2 and Donor 2 donates to Patient 1, allowing both patients to receive compatible kidneys.

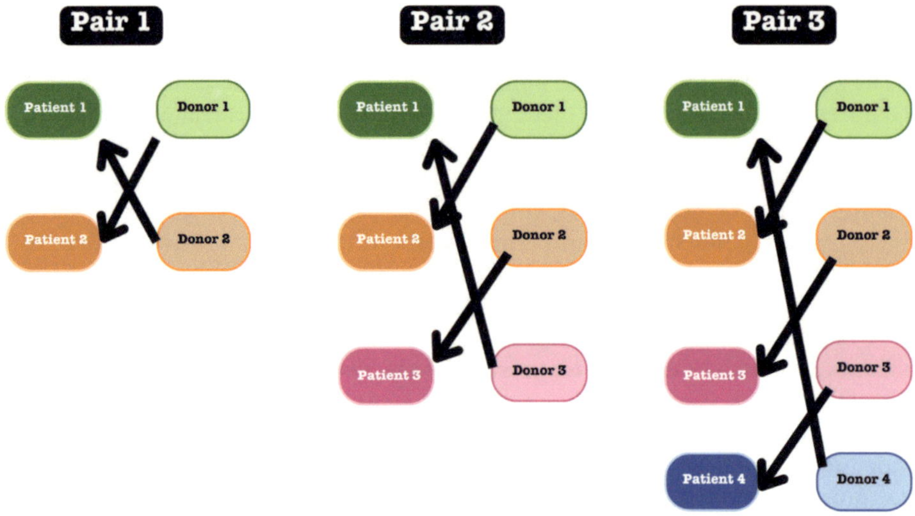

Figure 3.
An illustration of kidney paired donation exchanges, showing two-way, three-way, and four-way exchanges, increasing the number of successful transplants.

means that donors do not necessarily have to give their kidney directly to the recipient of the donor who is giving a kidney to their intended recipient. Instead, through a larger pool, more suitable matches can be found across different pairs, optimizing compatibility and outcomes (**Figure 3**).

The Dutch program reported that the 3-way exchange increases match rates from 54–66% [22], making it the most optimal length of kidney-paired donation to achieve reasonable match rates and simultaneous kidney transplants, especially for newly starting single-center programs. Longer chains do not lead to significantly more kidney transplants and add logistical burdens on the transplant team, requiring stringent and careful coordination.

One of the important examples of the progression of kidney paired donation (KPD) programs is the experience of an Indian center. This center started with a basic 2-way loop in 2000 and, after 13 years of gaining experience and confidence, progressed to a 3-way loop [23]. By 2020, they had further advanced to conducting a 10-way loop. This gradual evolution underscores the growing sophistication and effectiveness of KPD programs, demonstrating how incremental advancements in complexity can significantly enhance transplant facilitation.

One of the concerns in kidney paired Donation (KPD) programs is the potential for donors to renege in the middle of a chain. However, an analysis of 1748 transplants facilitated by the National Kidney Registry (NKR) found that broken chains are uncommon [24].

4.2 Expanding KPD: key strategies

Relying solely on conventional kidney paired donation (KPD) limits the potential for successful transplants, especially for patients with complex incompatibilities. Traditional methods cannot fully address the challenges posed by highly sensitized patients and those with difficult blood types, such as blood group O recipients. Expanding KPD strategies is essential for increasing match rates, improving transplant outcomes, and maximizing the donor pool. By incorporating innovative approaches, such as desensitization, ABO-incompatible transplants, and altruistic donor chains, KPD programs can better meet diverse patient needs and reduce wait times.

4.2.1 Incorporating compatible pairs in KPD

Incorporating compatible pairs into kidney paired donation (KPD) programs has proven to be a transformative strategy to expand the donor pool and improve matching opportunities for difficult-to-transplant recipients. Compatible donor-recipient pairs, when included in KPD, significantly enhance the match rate for incompatible pairs, effectively addressing the challenge of balancing blood-type mismatches and sensitized recipients. Studies, such as those by Gentry et al. [25], have demonstrated that including compatible pairs can nearly double the match rates, highlighting the efficiency of this approach in optimizing donor-recipient matching.

Recipients in KPD programs involving compatible pairs often receive kidneys from younger and healthier donors, improving post-transplant outcomes. Research by Chipman et al. [26] and Basu et al. [27] has shown that recipients benefit from kidneys with better Living Kidney Donor Profile Index (LKDPI) scores compared to their original donors. This improvement in donor quality not only enhances the immediate post-transplant outcomes but also contributes to the long-term success of the transplant.

The inclusion of compatible pairs also helps address issues related to sensitization and infectious mismatches. For instance, many compatible pairs enter KPD to avoid cytomegalovirus (CMV) or Epstein-Barr virus (EBV) mismatches, successfully mitigating these risks. This approach ensures better immunological compatibility and reduces post-transplant complications related to infectious diseases, as studies from Bingaman et al. [28] demonstrated (**Figure 4**).

Despite the clear benefits, ethical and logistical considerations must be addressed to optimize the implementation of compatible pairs in KPD. Fortin et al. [29] found

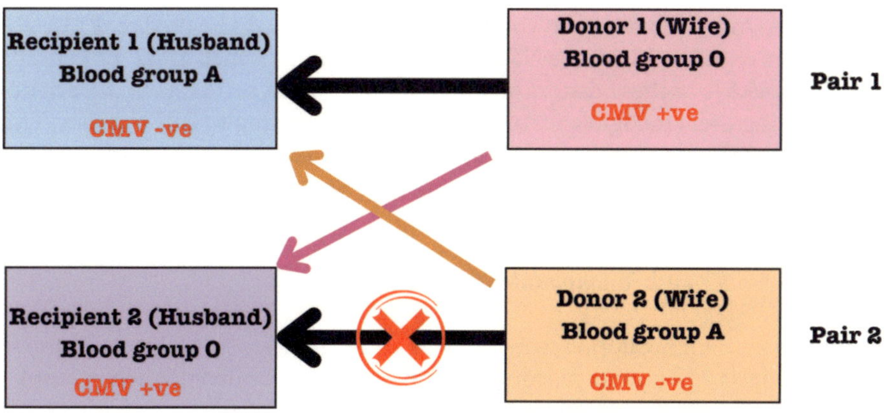

Figure 4.
This diagram illustrates a kidney paired donation (KPD) scenario involving two incompatible donor-recipient pairs. Recipient 1 (husband) and Donor 2 (wife) share compatibility in blood group A and CMV status, while Recipient 2 (husband) and Donor 1 (wife) share compatibility in blood group O and CMV status. The exchange allows both patients to receive kidneys from compatible donors, overcoming initial incompatibilities in their respective pairs.

that motivations for participation included the potential for optimal matching and policies ensuring prioritization for repeat transplantation. However, concerns about chain breaks, donor reneging, and delays in transplantation need systematic solutions. Overall, incorporating compatible pairs into KPD programs maximizes the potential of living donor kidney transplantation and provides equitable transplant opportunities for all patients.

4.2.2 A2 blood group in KPD

Blood group B candidates, especially among ethnic minorities, have historically faced significant barriers in accessing kidney transplantation, particularly in regions with a lower prevalence of blood group B [30]. Utilizing non-A1 kidneys, including the A2 subtype, has opened new opportunities for these patients. The A2 subtype expresses lower levels of A antigen on cell surfaces than the A1 subtype, making it less immunogenic and allowing it to act as a universal donor similar to blood group O [31].

A2 kidneys can be transplanted into blood type B and even O recipients using standard immunosuppression protocols, provided that the recipient's anti-A titers are sufficiently low. While most centers consider anti-A titers of less than 8 acceptable for transplantation [23], increasing this threshold to 16 could potentially expand the pool of eligible recipients, thereby improving access within KPD.

Studies on the long-term outcomes of A2 to O and B kidney transplants have demonstrated excellent graft survival rates comparable to those of ABO-compatible transplants. From 1986 through 2006, several blood group B and O patients received kidneys from blood group A2 donors. The data showed that graft survival rates for B recipients of A2/A2B kidneys were equivalent to those for B recipients of B kidneys.

A2 kidneys have already started to be utilized in the kidney allocation system (KAS) for deceased donors; incorporating them into KPD could further enhance the effectiveness and reach of these programs.

The accuracy of subtyping is crucial in ensuring that A2 donors are correctly identified and utilized. Between February 2018 and September 2020, the National Kidney Registry (NKR) performed serological typing on all A/AB donors and confirmed non-A1/non-A1B donors through genotyping. They discovered that 13.0% of type A donors registered with the NKR were ultimately subtyped as A2 via genotyping. Notably, 49.6% of these donors had initially been subtyped as A1 at their donor centers, making them ineligible for allocation as A2 according to OPTN policy. This inaccuracy represents a significant lost opportunity in transplantation, especially in KPD, where A2 donors can facilitate additional living donor transplants and benefit highly sensitized candidates.

4.2.3 KPD combined with incompatible ABO transplantation

Advances in immunosuppressive protocols and antibody removal techniques, such as plasmapheresis and immunoadsorption, have made ABO-incompatible transplants more feasible. These methods allow patients with low to moderate anti-blood group antibody (ABGAb) titers to receive kidneys from ABO-incompatible donors, achieving outcomes comparable to those of ABO-compatible transplants. This approach is particularly beneficial in kidney-paired donation (KPD) programs, where combining KPD with ABO-incompatible transplants can further expand the pool of available donors, thereby increasing the number of successful transplants.

For example, a patient-donor pairs with high ABO titers [pair 1: patient 1 (O group) and donor 1 (A group) with an anti-A isoagglutinin titer >512; pair 2: patient 2 (O group) and donor 2 (B group) with an anti-B isoagglutinin titer >512] can exchange kidneys to receive a donor with low ABO titers [pair 1: patient 1 (O group) and donor 2 (B group) with an anti-B isoagglutinin titer <64; pair 2: patient 2 (O group) and donor 1 (A group) with an anti-A isoagglutinin titer <64]. This strategy minimizes costs, reduces the need for intensive immunosuppression, and enhances long-term outcomes for ABO-incompatible kidney transplantation while increasing match rates for sensitized patients. Studies have shown that ABO-incompatible transplantation, in the absence of donor-specific antibodies and with low baseline ABO titers (< 1:64), has good outcomes (**Figure 5**).

Integrating ABO incompatibility solutions within KPD programs enhances their flexibility and efficacy. By including ABO-incompatible pairs, KPD programs can form more extensive and complex chains, optimizing the use of available donors and expanding the pool of compatible recipients. This approach maximizes transplant opportunities and addresses disparities in access to transplantation, particularly benefiting highly sensitized patients. The Australian KPD program's success in accepting ABO-incompatible donors [32], which resulted in a significant increase in transplant rates, demonstrates the potential of such integrated strategies to improve the effectiveness and reach of KPD programs globally.

4.2.4 Desensitization combinations

Desensitization has shown good outcomes when starting donor-specific antibody strength is low. For broadly sensitized patients with a high-strength cross-match, a better donor can often be found in a KPD pool, facilitating safer and more successful desensitization [33].

Combining kidney-paired donation (KPD) with desensitization strategies significantly enhances transplant rates for highly sensitized patients. These patients often face substantial barriers to finding compatible donors due to ABO or HLA

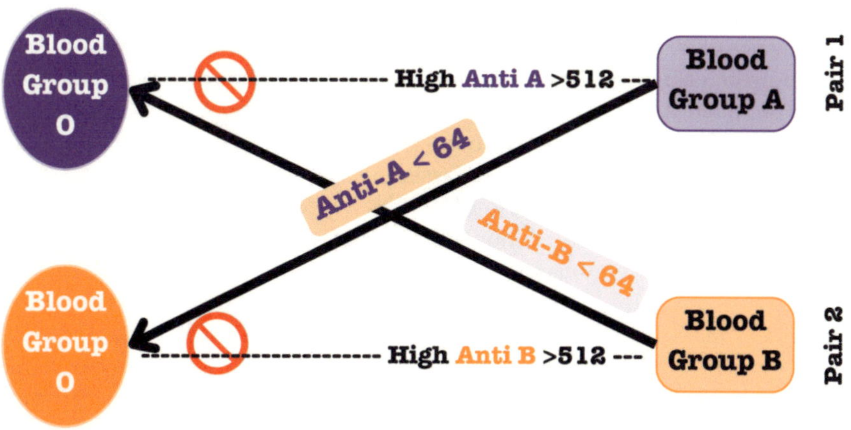

Figure 5.
The figure shows a blood group-based kidney exchange between two incompatible pairs. Pair 1 involves a patient with blood group O and high anti-A titers (>512) receiving a kidney from Pair 2's donor with blood group B and low anti-B titers (<64). Simultaneously, Pair 2's patient with blood group O and high anti-B titers (>512) receives a kidney from Pair 1's donor with blood group A and low anti-A titers (<64). This exchange enables successful transplantation without extensive desensitization.

incompatibilities. The integration of desensitization protocols with KPD broadens the pool of potential donors, particularly benefiting those with high calculated panel-reactive antibody (cPRA) levels. This combined approach has shown a 66% increase in transplant rates, addressing the critical issue of long wait times for highly sensitized patients [34].

Sensitized patients comprise 30% of the kidney transplant waiting list, yet fewer than 15% of highly sensitized patients are transplanted each year. Traditional options for these patients include desensitization or KPD, but these methods alone may not be sufficient for recipients with cumulative cPRA >95%. Combining both approaches maximizes the likelihood of finding a compatible match with a more immunologically favorable donor through a kidney exchange program. This combined approach was successfully used in five highly sensitized patients, all with cPRA 100%, who received compatible living and deceased donor kidney transplants [35].

The integration of KPD with desensitization protocols has become increasingly common, particularly for highly sensitized patients. In a study of 170 kidney recipients transplanted by KPD, 75 received concomitant desensitization. The outcomes of KPD combined with desensitization were comparable to those of compatible transplants. Kaplan–Meier estimates showed no significant difference in patient survival, death-censored graft survival, and overall graft survival between the two strategies [36]. This demonstrates that incompatible pairs, which do not benefit from KPD or desensitization alone, achieve similar outcomes when both modalities are combined.

4.2.5 Altruistic chains: NDAD and NEAD

Incorporating altruistic donors, often called "Good Samaritans," "anonymous", or "benevolent community donors", into kidney-paired donation (KPD) systems significantly enhances the potential for successful transplants. Altruistic donors are individuals who donate a kidney without a designated recipient, motivated purely by the desire to help someone needing a transplant. Their contributions can initiate a "Domino Effect" within the KPD framework, where a single altruistic donation sets off a chain of transplants, exponentially increasing the number of recipients who can benefit.

One of the pioneering reports [37] of such a chain in the United States documented a series of 10 transplants initiated by a single altruistic donor in July 2007. This chain, which concluded in 2009, involved six transplantation centers across five states and included simultaneous and non-simultaneous surgeries. Notably, 6 of the 10 recipients had a panel reactive antibody (PRA) level greater than 60%, highlighting the effectiveness of this approach in assisting highly sensitized patients.

In the non-directed altruistic donor (NDAD) model, a non-directed donor starts a sequence where each recipient's donor subsequently donates to the following recipient in the chain, potentially ending with a donation to the waitlist. An advancement of this model is the non-simultaneous extended altruistic donor (NEAD) chain, where the final donor in the sequence, known as a bridge donor, waits to initiate another chain, thus creating a continuous cycle of donations. Since 2008, kidney exchange in America has grown significantly due to the incorporation of non-directed donors in transplant chains rather than simple exchanges. It is controversial whether these chains should be performed simultaneously as "domino-paired donation" (DPD) or non-simultaneously as NEAD chains. NEAD chains create "bridge donors" whose incompatible recipients receive kidneys before the bridge donor donates, risking reneging by bridge donors, but offering the opportunity to create more transplants by overcoming logistical barriers inherent in simultaneous chains [38].

Gentry et al. [37] conducted simulations to compare the effectiveness of domino-paired donation (DPD) and non-simultaneous extended altruistic donor (NEAD) chains in producing transplants. When limiting the chain segment length to three transplants, their findings showed that DPD performed as well as NEAD chains. However, this contrasts with the experiences of several kidney-paired donation groups. Simulations that allowed for longer chain segments (4–6 transplants) and used real patient data from the Alliance for Paired Donation demonstrated that NEAD chains resulted in more transplants than DPD. Additionally, NEAD chains were particularly effective in producing transplants for highly sensitized and blood type O recipients.

Altruistic donor chains, particularly those initiated by donors with blood type O, have proven exceptionally beneficial. A study involving 77 non-directed donors demonstrated that these donors-initiated chains averaging nearly five transplants each, with blood type O donors facilitating even longer chains [39]. Additionally, a multicenter study [40] involving 16 transplant centers showed that 70 domino chains initiated by altruistic donors resulted in 179 kidney transplants, with impressive one-year and five-year graft survival rates of 98.3% and 87.7%, respectively. These chains are crucial for matching highly sensitized patients and those with blood type O, who typically face longer wait times.

In a list exchange (LE), an intended recipient in an incompatible pair receives priority on the deceased donor waitlist after their paired incompatible donor gives a kidney to a waitlist candidate, thus optimizing the transplant process [41]. Similarly, incorporating deceased donor (DD) kidneys to initiate transplant chains within a KPD pool has been shown to increase the number of transplants by at least 447 over two years (**Figure 6**) [42].

However, incorporating altruistic donors into KPD systems also presents challenges. The NEAD model, for instance, often faces difficulties with AB blood type bridge

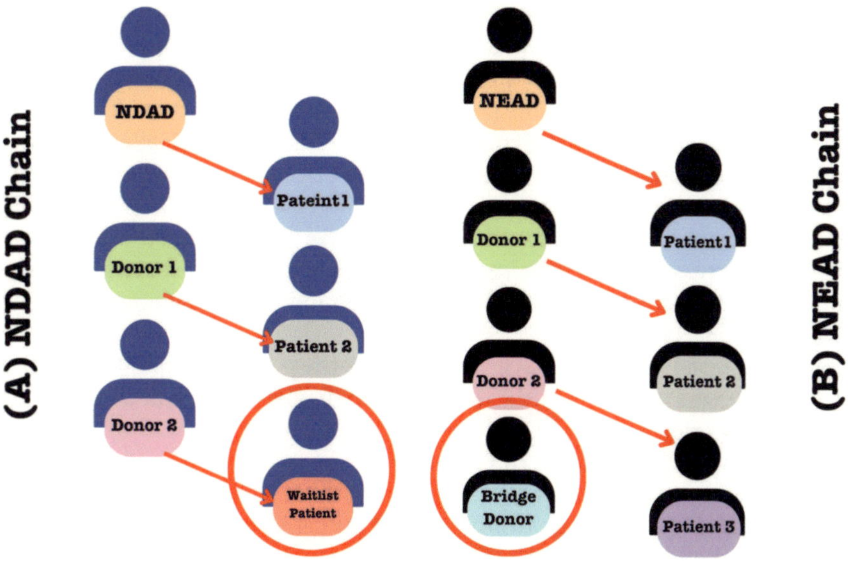

Figure 6.
This diagram compares two kidney paired donation chain strategies. In (A) the NDAD chain, an altruistic non-directed donor initiates the chain, with the final donor in the sequence donating to a patient on the waitlist. In (B) the NEAD chain, an altruistic donor starts the chain, but the final donor becomes a bridge donor, creating potential for further transplants in subsequent chains. Both strategies aim to maximize transplant opportunities, but NEAD chains extend the chain's impact over time.

donors due to the smaller pool of compatible recipients, which can lead to prolonged waiting periods and an increased risk of bridge donors reneging. Despite these challenges, simulations have shown that NEAD chains can result in more transplants compared to traditional simultaneous domino-paired donations [43].

The flexibility and potential for extended chains make the incorporation of altruistic donors a vital strategy in KPD. These chains not only increase the number of transplants but also optimize the use of available donors, leading to improved outcomes for a broader set of recipients. By expanding the donor pool and facilitating complex matching scenarios, altruistic donors play a pivotal role in addressing the organ shortage crisis and enhancing the effectiveness of kidney paired donation programs.

5. Expanding horizons in kidney paired donation

5.1 International KPD

International kidney paired donation (IKPD) offers a promising avenue to expand the donor pool and improve matching opportunities on a global scale. This approach not only addresses biological incompatibilities but also bridges financial barriers, facilitating transplants for patients across both high-income and low- to middle-income countries. By connecting donor-recipient pairs from different countries, international KPD leverages the diverse genetic pool and varying availability of donors globally, thus increasing the chances of finding suitable matches for highly sensitized patients or those with rare blood types [44].

One notable initiative in this domain is the Global Kidney Exchange (GKE), which aims to overcome financial incompatibilities that often prevent transplants in lower-income countries. GKE involves entering international pairs into a US-based kidney exchange program, which provides long-term financial support and facilitates suitable exchanges for both international pairs and US citizens. The first GKE transplant, conducted with a Filipino husband and wife, successfully provided a kidney for the husband while integrating the couple into a non-simultaneous extended altruistic chain, benefiting multiple recipients in the United States [45]. Furthermore, the first international KPD transplantation from India involved a two-way kidney exchange between pairs from Portugal and India. This initiative underscored the feasibility and benefits of cross-border exchanges, particularly for highly sensitized and ABO-incompatible patients. Both pairs underwent simultaneous transplant surgeries with successful outcomes [46].

However, international KPD faces criticism for the potential exploitation of financially disadvantaged donors, healthcare inequities in post-transplant care, and the risk of diverting resources from developing local transplant programs. Ethical concerns include ensuring voluntary and informed consent and managing the disparity in healthcare standards across countries. Addressing these challenges through stringent ethical guidelines, equitable care protocols, and robust international agreements can help mitigate risks and enhance the efficacy of international KPD programs.

5.2 Trans-organ exchange (liver-kidney exchange)

Trans-organ paired exchange is an innovative concept that expands the potential for organ donation by allowing donors who are unsuitable for donating one organ to contribute to the transplant system by donating another organ. This approach enables donors who may be ruled out for kidney-specific reasons to donate a liver and vice versa. For instance [47], a person with a mild reduction in glomerular filtration rate (GFR) or complex kidney anatomy may be ruled out as a kidney donor but can still be a viable liver donor. Conversely, a potential liver donor with aberrant liver anatomy might be a suitable kidney donor.

To date, only a few trans-organ paired exchanges have been reported. One notable case [48] involved a 19-year-old who was ruled out as a kidney donor but requested to donate her liver in exchange for a kidney for her mother, who had end-stage renal disease (ESRD). This pair was matched with another donor-recipient pair where the potential liver donor had an anatomical issue precluding liver donation but was suitable for kidney donation. Despite initial donor incompatibilities, this swap enabled both recipients to receive the needed organs.

Trans-organ paired exchange raises several ethical and legal questions. The National Organ Transplant Act (NOTA) allows for organ-paired donation but does not specify that the organs must be the same, making trans-organ exchanges legally permissible. However, ethical concerns include the disparity in risk between kidney and liver donations. Kidney donation carries a mortality risk of approximately 1 in 3000, while liver donation's risk is about 1 in 500. Additionally, liver donors face a longer recovery period and more immediate postoperative risks compared to kidney donors. Ensuring that donors provide informed and voluntary consent is crucial. Potential donors must understand the differential risks and benefits involved, and transplant teams must protect donors from coercion and ensure they have the opportunity to withdraw consent without feeling undue pressure.

6. Criteria for KPD entry and advanced algorithms and software

The criteria for kidney paired donation (KPD) include HLA incompatibility, ABO incompatibility, significant age differences (more than 10 years if the donor is under 50), size mismatch (donor's Iothalamate GFR corrected for recipient's body surface area divided by 2 is less than 35), CMV/EBV mismatch, and altruistic reasons [27].

As KPD programs evolve, the number of potential donor-recipient combinations grows exponentially, presenting a significant mathematical challenge. This graph illustrates how combinations increase as more pairs participate. With 100 pairs, potential matches are relatively small, but approaching 500 pairs, combinations skyrocket to tens of thousands. To manage this complexity, advanced algorithmic software designed for organ matching is utilized. This software inputs each participant's medical data, including blood type, tissue compatibility, and immunological factors, to generate compatibility scores for every possible pair.

Modern KPD programs significantly benefit from integrating advanced algorithms and sophisticated software. These innovations optimize the matching process, ensuring efficient and accurate pairings between donors and recipients. The software used in KPD registries manages and analyzes vast amounts of data, incorporating immunological data, such as HLA typing and crossmatch results to create compatibility matrices. By assigning point scores to potential matches, the software generates optimized solutions, efficiently identifying the best donor-recipient pairings. Advanced algorithms and software optimize both closed-loop conventional exchanges and chain strategies based on the likelihood of better transplants, prioritizing sensitized recipients, avoiding viral mismatches, and focusing on chain length for maximum efficiency.

Additionally, KPD guidelines emphasize that less compatible kidneys should never be offered. Pre-emptive transplantation is prioritized, especially if the recipient is near needing dialysis, and decisions are re-evaluated every three months. ABO/HLA compatible pairs always have the option to proceed directly to transplantation outside of KPD.

Centralized databases and real-time updates in the software enable seamless coordination between multiple transplant centers, minimizing delays, and improving overall process efficiency. For instance, the Alliance for Paired Donation (APD) [49] uses a web-based virtual matching system that has evolved over seven years to improve conversion rates from computer-identified matches to successful transplants. This system not only proposes optimal matches but also helps track and manage offers, perform crossmatches, and handle logistical details effectively.

In practical application, advanced algorithmic software dynamically adapts to changes such as new pairs joining the pool or updates in a recipient's medical condition, ensuring the matching process remains efficient and adaptable. For example, with 10 incompatible pairs, arranging them into a single chain could potentially facilitate up to seven transplants if all goes perfectly. However, this is often not the most efficient or feasible scenario due to various compatibility and logistical challenges. With sophisticated algorithmic software, alternative arrangements can be explored to increase the total number of successful transplants. The software might suggest splitting the 10 pairs into two shorter chains or loops, maximizing the use of available donors and enhancing the chances for patients to receive transplants faster and with better matches.

In summary, the software does not just seek to match pairs—it aims to optimize the entire system to maximize successful transplants. It creates multiple chains and loops, ensuring that as many patients as possible receive the kidneys they need. The dynamic nature of the software allows it to adapt to changes, such as new pairs joining the pool or updates in a recipient's medical condition, ensuring the matching process remains efficient and adaptable (**Figure 7**).

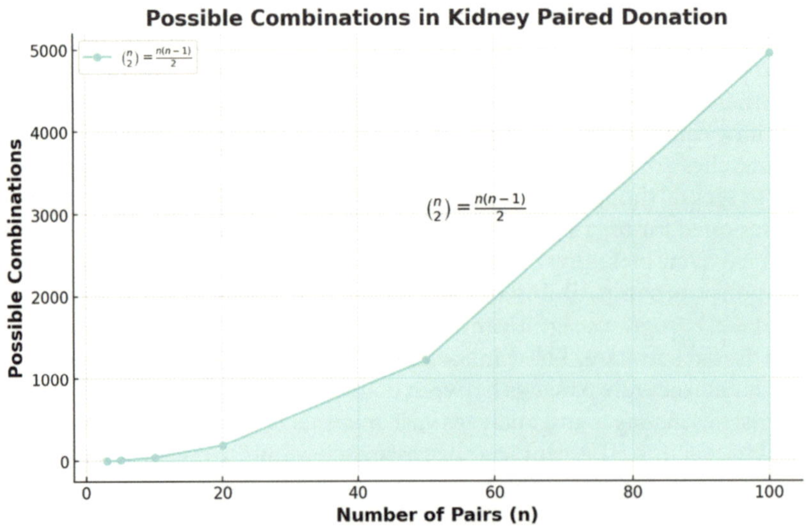

Figure 7.
Graph showing the exponential increase in possible combinations as the number of pairs in a kidney-paired donation program increases, illustrating the complexity and potential of matching algorithms in such programs.

7. Ethical challenges in KPD programs

Kidney-paired donation (KPD) programs face numerous ethical challenges [50], primarily ensuring equitable access to kidney transplants. Socioeconomic disparities often hinder fair access, especially for individuals in poverty or without medical insurance. Addressing these financial and logistical barriers is crucial for ethical integrity. Additionally, maintaining donor autonomy is vital, requiring comprehensive informed consent and clear communication about the risks and implications involved in the donation process.

Another significant challenge is safeguarding patient data, ensuring privacy, and protection against unauthorized access. Balancing financial incentives to support donors while preventing organ commercialization is also critical. Furthermore, managing expectations and preparing patients and families for potential negative outcomes through thorough counseling and support is essential. Logistical issues, such as ensuring donor anonymity, addressing concerns about age differences and kidney quality, and coordinating simultaneous operations to prevent donor reneging, are integral to the program's ethical success.

8. Key requirements and strategies for implementing a successful KPD program

Establishing a successful kidney-paired donation (KPD) program involves several critical components. Firstly, a robust KPD registry is essential for efficiently tracking participants and outcomes. Uniform evaluations and care protocols across all facilities ensure consistent and fair treatment. Standardizing HLA laboratory testing is crucial for accurate donor-recipient matching. Ensuring similar quality kidneys are exchanged maintains equity in transplantation outcomes. Simultaneous surgeries prevent donors from withdrawing post-nephrectomy of the recipient. Finally, a non-anonymous allocation process enhances transparency and trust among participants.

The strategy for developing a kidney-paired exchange (KPE) program [48] emphasizes gradual growth, starting with centralization and standardization. Establishing a National Transplant Centre is central to this strategy, coordinating all components of the KPE program and facilitating improved collaboration between healthcare sectors. Standardizing protocols for preparing donors and recipients simplifies the exchange process and sets a foundation for future expansion.

Building community confidence through adherence to high ethical standards is crucial, aligning with international principles on organ donation and transplantation. Robust legal frameworks must protect participants and prevent organ trafficking. Engaging public opinion and gaining stakeholder consensus are critical steps in this phase. This foundational work ensures the KPE program operates with integrity and public trust.

Continuous monitoring through analysis of transplant rates, graft survival, and patient quality of life provides crucial insights into the program's effectiveness. As the National Transplant Centre gains experience, particularly with simpler 2-way exchanges, the program can strategically expand to more complex exchange types. This methodical expansion ensures the program remains adaptable and scalable, maintaining high-quality service without compromising the integrity or outcomes of the exchanges. By continuously evaluating and refining the process, the KPE program can achieve sustainable growth and success.

Acknowledgements

The authors extend their gratitude to Yasmeen Jamal Alabdallat, a distinguished student at Hashemite University, for her invaluable assistance in creating the figures and diagrams presented in this work.

Appendices and nomenclature

KPD (Kidney paired donation)	A transplant option where incompatible donor-recipient pairs are matched with other pairs in similar situations to enable kidney exchanges
NDAD (Non-directed altruistic donor)	An individual who donates a kidney without a designated recipient, often initiating a chain of transplants
cPRA (Calculated panel reactive antibody)	A measure of a patient's sensitization to potential donors, expressed as a percentage

Author details

Mohammad Hassan Al-thnaibat
Hashemite University, Zarqa, Jordan

*Address all correspondence to: moh1.thunibat@gmail.com

References

[1] Tonelli M, Wiebe N, Knoll G, Bello A, Browne S, Jadhav D, et al. Systematic review: Kidney transplantation compared with dialysis in clinically relevant outcomes. American Journal of Transplantation. 2011;**11**(10):2093-2109. DOI: 10.1111/j.1600-6143.2011.03686.x

[2] International Registry in Organ Donation and Transplantation International Registry in Organ Donation and Transplantation. Available from: https://www.irodat.org/

[3] Nemati E, Einollahi B, Lesan Pezeshki M, Porfarziani V, Fattahi MR. Does kidney transplantation with deceased or living donor affect graft survival? Nephro-Urology Monthly. 2014;**6**(4):e12182. DOI: 10.5812/numonthly.12182

[4] Salas MAP, Chua E, Rossi A, Shah S, Katz-Greenberg G, Coscia L, et al. Sex and gender disparity in kidney transplantation: Historical and future perspectives. Clinical Transplantation. 2022;**36**(12):e14814. DOI: 10.1111/ctr.14814

[5] Al-Thnaibat MH, Balaw MK, Al-Aquily MK, Ghannam RA, Mohd OB, Alabidi F, et al. Addressing kidney transplant shortage: The potential of kidney paired exchanges in Jordan. Journal of Transplantation. 2024;**2024**:4538034. DOI: 10.1155/2024/4538034

[6] Jackson KR, Motter JD, Kernodle A, Desai N, Thomas AG, Massie AB, et al. How do highly sensitized patients get kidney transplants in the United States? Trends over the last decade. American Journal of Transplantation. 2020;**20**(8):2101-2112. DOI: 10.1111/ajt.15825

[7] Keith DS, Vranic GM. Approach to the highly sensitized kidney transplant candidate. Clinical Journal of the American Society of Nephrology. 2016;**11**(4):684-693. DOI: 10.2215/CJN.05930615

[8] Etxebarria A, Díez-Martín E, Astigarraga E, Barreda-Gómez G. Role of the immune system in renal transplantation, types of response, technical approaches and current challenges. Immuno. 2022;**2**:548-570. DOI: 10.3390/immuno2040035

[9] Glander P, Budde K, Schmidt D, Fuller TF, Giessing M, Neumayer HH, et al. The 'blood group O problem' in kidney transplantation--time to change? Nephrology, Dialysis, Transplantation. 2010;**25**(6):1998-2004. DOI: 10.1093/ndt/gfp779

[10] Wallis CB, Samy KP, Roth AE, Rees MA. Kidney paired donation. Nephrology, Dialysis, Transplantation. 2011;**26**(7):2091-2099. DOI: 10.1093/ndt/gfr155

[11] Abu Jawdeh BG, Cuffy MC, Alloway RR, Shields AR, Woodle ES. Desensitization in kidney transplantation: Review and future perspectives. Clinical Transplantation. 2014;**28**(4):494-507. DOI: 10.1111/ctr.12335

[12] Marfo K, Lu A, Ling M, Akalin E. Desensitization protocols and their outcome. Clinical Journal of the American Society of Nephrology. 2011;**6**(4):922-936. DOI: 10.2215/CJN.08140910

[13] Schinstock C, Tambur A, Stegall M. Current approaches to desensitization in solid organ transplantation. Frontiers

in Immunology. 2021;**12**:686271. DOI: 10.3389/fimmu.2021.686271

[14] Rapaport FT. The case for a living emotionally related international kidney donor exchange registry. Transplantation Proceedings. 1986;**18**((3) Suppl. 2):5-9

[15] Kwak JY, Kwon OJ, Lee KS, Kang CM, Park HY, Kim JH. Exchange-donor program in renal transplantation: A single-center experience. Transplantation Proceedings. 1999;**31**(1-2):344-345. DOI: 10.1016/s0041-1345(98)01655-8

[16] de Klerk M, Keizer KM, Claas FH, Witvliet M, Haase-Kromwijk BJ, Weimar W. The Dutch national living donor kidney exchange program. American Journal of Transplantation. 2005;**5**(9):2302-2305. DOI: 10.1111/j.1600-6143.2005.01024.x

[17] Hadaya K, Fehr T, Rüsi B, Ferrari-Lacraz S, Jean V, Ferrari P. Kidney paired donation: A plea for a Swiss National Programme. Swiss Medical Weekly. 2015;**145**:w14083. DOI: 10.4414/smw.2015.14083

[18] Cole EH, Nickerson P, Campbell P, Yetzer K, Lahaie N, Zaltzman J, et al. The Canadian kidney paired donation program: A national program to increase living donor transplantation. Transplantation. 2015;**99**(5):985-990. DOI: 10.1097/TP.0000000000000455

[19] Cantwell L, Woodroffe C, Holdsworth R, Ferrari P. Four years of experience with the Australian kidney paired donation programme. Nephrology (Carlton, Vic.). 2015;**20**(3):124-131. DOI: 10.1111/nep.12369

[20] Leopold SS. A conversation with ... Alvin E. Roth PhD, economist, game theorist, and Nobel laureate who improved the modern residency match. Clinical Orthopaedics and Related Research. 2021;**479**(5):863-866. DOI: 10.1097/CORR.0000000000001758

[21] Glorie K, Haase-Kromwijk B, van de Klundert J, Wagelmans A, Weimar W. Allocation and matching in kidney exchange programs. Transplant International. 2014;**27**(4):333-343. DOI: 10.1111/tri.12202. Epub 2013 Oct 17

[22] Saidman SL, Roth AE, Sönmez T, Unver MU, Delmonico FL. Increasing the opportunity of live kidney donation by matching for two- and three-way exchanges. Transplantation. 2006;**81**(5):773-782. DOI: 10.1097/01.tp.0000195775.77081.25

[23] Kute VB, Patel HV, Shah PR, Modi PR, Shah VR, Rizvi SJ, et al. Past, present and future of kidney paired donation transplantation in India. World Journal of Transplantation. 2017;**7**(2):134-143. DOI: 10.5500/wjt.v7.i2.134

[24] Cowan N, Gritsch HA, Nassiri N, Sinacore J, Veale J. Broken chains and reneging: A review of 1748 kidney paired donation transplants. American Journal of Transplantation. 2017;**17**(9):2451-2457. DOI: 10.1111/ajt.14343

[25] Gentry SE, Segev DL, Simmerling M, Montgomery RA. Expanding kidney paired donation through participation by compatible pairs. American Journal of Transplantation. 2007;**7**(10):2361-2370. DOI: 10.1111/j.1600-6143.2007.01935.x

[26] Chipman V, Cooper M, Thomas AG, Ronin M, Lee B, Flechner S, et al. Motivations and outcomes of compatible living donor-recipient pairs in paired exchange. American Journal of Transplantation. 2022;**22**(1):266-273. DOI: 10.1111/ajt.16821

[27] Basu A, Prieto M, Kosberg C, Mai ML, Khamash HA, Jadlowiec CC,

et al. Ten years of kidney paired donation at Mayo Clinic: The benefits of incorporating ABO/HLA compatible pairs. Transplantation. 2020;**104**(6):1229-1238. DOI: 10.1097/TP.0000000000002947

[28] Bingaman A, Wright F, Kapturczak M, Shen L, Murphey C. Utilization of compatible pairs in a large kidney paired donation program [abstract]. 2013 American Transplant Congress (ATC meeting). American Journal of Transplantation. 2013;**13**(suppl. 5). Abstract number: 566. Available from: https://atcmeetingabstracts.com/abstract/utilization-of-compatible-pairs-in-a-large-kidney-paired-donation-program/ [Accessed: June 18, 2024]

[29] Fortin MC, Gill J, Allard J, Ballesteros Gallego F, Gill J. Compatible donor and recipient Pairs' perspectives on participation in kidney paired donation programs: A mixed-methods study. Canadian Journal of Kidney Health and Disease. 2021;**8**:20543581211058932. DOI: 10.1177/20543581211058932

[30] Gloor JM, Lager DJ, Moore SB, Pineda AA, Fidler ME, Larson TS, et al. ABO-incompatible kidney transplantation using both A2 and non-A2 living donors. Transplantation. 2003;**75**(7):971-977. DOI: 10.1097/01.TP.0000058226.39732.32

[31] Williams WW, Cherikh WS, Young CJ, Fan PY, Cheng Y, Distant DA, et al. First report on the OPTN National Variance: Allocation of A2/A2 B deceased donor kidneys to blood group B increases minority transplantation. American Journal of Transplantation. 2015;**15**(12):3134-3142. DOI: 10.1111/ajt.13409

[32] Ferrari P, Hughes PD, Cohney SJ, Woodroffe C, Fidler S, D'Orsogna L. ABO-incompatible matching significantly enhances transplant rates in kidney paired donation. Transplantation. 2013;**96**(9):821-826. DOI: 10.1097/TP.0b013e3182a01311

[33] Montgomery RA, Lonze BE, Jackson AM. Using donor exchange paradigms with desensitization to enhance transplant rates among highly sensitized patients. Current Opinion in Organ Transplantation. 2011;**16**(4):439-443. DOI: 10.1097/MOT.0b013e32834897c1

[34] Pham TA, Lee JI, Melcher ML. Kidney paired exchange and desensitization: Strategies to transplant the difficult to match kidney patients with living donors. Transplantation Reviews (Orlando, Fla.). 2017;**31**(1):29-34. DOI: 10.1016/j.trre.2017.01.003

[35] Yabu JM, Pando MJ, Busque S, Melcher ML. Desensitization combined with paired exchange leads to successful transplantation in highly sensitized kidney transplant recipients: Strategy and report of five cases. Transplantation Proceedings. 2013;**45**(1):82-87. DOI: 10.1016/j.transproceed.2012.08.007

[36] Sharif A, Lonze B, Hillier J, Zachary A, Leffell M, Alachkar N, et al. Outcomes from combining kidney paired donation and desensitization: An approach to kidney transplantation for the Most highly sensitized patients: 2474. Transplantation. 2012;**94**(10S):83

[37] Gentry SE, Montgomery RA, Swihart BJ, Segev DL. The roles of dominos and nonsimultaneous chains in kidney paired donation. American Journal of Transplantation. 2009;**9**(6):1330-1336. DOI: 10.1111/j.1600-6143.2009.02622.x

[38] Ashlagi I, Gilchrist DS, Roth AE, Rees MA. Nonsimultaneous chains and dominos in kidney-paired

donation—Revisited. American Journal of Transplantation. 2011;**11**(5):984-994. DOI: 10.1111/j.1600-6143.2011.03481.x

[39] Melcher ML, Veale JL, Javaid B, Leeser DB, Davis CL, Hil G, et al. Kidney transplant chains amplify benefit of nondirected donors. JAMA Surgery. 2013;**148**(2):165-170. DOI: 10.1001/2013.jamasurg.25

[40] Lee YJ, Lee SU, Chung SY, Cho BH, Kwak JY, Kang CM, et al. Clinical outcomes of multicenter domino kidney paired donation. American Journal of Transplantation. 2009;**9**(10):2424-2428. DOI: 10.1111/j.1600-6143.2009.02747.x

[41] Roth AE, Sönmez T, Unver MU, Delmonico FL, Saidman SL. Utilizing list exchange and nondirected donation through 'chain' paired kidney donations. American Journal of Transplantation. 2006;**6**(11):2694-2705. DOI: 10.1111/j.1600-6143.2006.01515.x

[42] Wang W, Rees MA, Leichtman AB, Song PX, Bray M, Ashby VB, et al. Deceased donors as nondirected donors in kidney paired donation. American Journal of Transplantation. 2021;**21**(1):103-113. DOI: 10.1111/ajt.16268

[43] Blumberg JM, Gritsch H, Veale JL. Kidney paired donation: Advancements and future directions. Current Opinion in Organ Transplantation. 2011;**16**(4):418-423. DOI: 10.1097/MOT.0b013e328348bfe2

[44] Rees MA, Paloyo SR, Roth AE, Krawiec KD, Ekwenna O, Marsh CL, et al. Global kidney exchange: Financially incompatible pairs are not transplantable compatible pairs. American Journal of Transplantation. 2017;**17**(10):2743-2744. DOI: 10.1111/ajt.14451

[45] Bozek DN, Dunn TB, Kuhr CS, Marsh CL, Rogers J, Rees SE, et al. Complete chain of the first global kidney exchange transplant and 3-yr follow-up. European Urology Focus. 2018;**4**(2):190-197. DOI: 10.1016/j.euf.2018.07.021

[46] Kute VB, Patel HV, Shah PR, Modi PR, Shah VR, Rizvi SJ, et al. International kidney paired donation transplantations to increase kidney transplant of O group and highly sensitized patient: First report from India. World Journal of Transplantation. 2017;**7**(1):64-69. DOI: 10.5500/wjt.v7.i1.64

[47] Samstein B, de Melo-Martin I, Kapur S, Ratner L, Emond J. A liver for a kidney: Ethics of trans-organ paired exchange. American Journal of Transplantation. 2018;**18**(5):1077-1082. DOI: 10.1111/ajt.14690

[48] Torres AM, Wong F, Pearson S, Weinberg S, Roberts JP, Ascher NL, et al. Bi-organ paired exchange-sentinel case of a liver-kidney swap. American Journal of Transplantation. 2019;**19**(9):2646-2649. DOI: 10.1111/ajt.15386

[49] Fumo DE, Kapoor V, Reece LJ, Stepkowski SM, Kopke JE, Rees SE, et al. Historical matching strategies in kidney paired donation: The 7-year evolution of a web-based virtual matching system. American Journal of Transplantation. 2015;**15**(10):2646-2654. DOI: 10.1111/ajt.13337. Epub 2015 May 26

[50] Patel SR, Chadha P, Papalois V. Expanding the live kidney donor pool: Ethical considerations regarding altruistic donors, paired and pooled programs. Experimental and Clinical Transplantation. 2011;**9**(3):181-186

Chapter 5

Complement Activation in Kidney Transplantation

Pande Made Wisnu Tirtayasa, Gerhard Reinaldi Situmorang, Gede Wirya Kusuma Duarsa, Arry Rodjani and Nur Rasyid

Abstract

Kidney transplantation is a life-saving procedure for individuals with end-stage renal disease, yet the process of transplantation can trigger the activation of the complement system, a critical component of the body's immune response. This activation can lead to adverse outcomes, including acute and chronic rejection of the graft, thereby complicating patient management and graft survival. Furthermore, the interplay between complement activation and immunosuppressive therapies remains a key area of research, as prolonged immunosuppression may enhance the risk of complications while failing to adequately control the immune response against the transplanted organ, necessitating a balance between these factors to optimize transplant outcomes. In recent years, advances in understanding the mechanisms of complement activation have led to the exploration of novel therapeutic strategies aimed at minimizing damage to the graft and enhancing its long-term functionality, emphasizing the need for tailored immunosuppressive regimens to mitigate the associated risks and improve the overall success of kidney transplantation.

Keywords: kidney transplant, immunology, complement activation, allograft rejection, immunosuppression

1. Introduction

The domain of organ transplantation experiences notable progression over durations, though challenges persist, notably within the domain of immunological reactions, which may result in graft rejection. Complement activation, an essential element of the innate immune system, has appeared as a significant factor in the series of incidents that decisively influence the fate of transplanted organs. Within the context of kidney transplantation, complement activation could be instigated by numerous factors, encompassing ischemia-reperfusion injury, donor-specific antibodies, and immune complexes formed after transplantation. Comprehending the detailed interaction between complement activation and the adaptive immune response presents substantial potential for ameliorating outcomes in kidney transplantation. By decoding the elaborate mechanisms underpinning complement activation within this context, new therapeutic approaches may be conceived to augment graft survival and prolonged functioning, thereby ultimately profiting transplant recipients.

IntechOpen

1.1 Background of kidney transplantation

Kidney transplantation represents a crucial medical intervention for individuals experiencing end-stage renal disease (ESRD), contributing significantly toward saving lives. The inception of kidney transplantation as a medical practice can be traced back to the mid-twentieth century, a period marked by enhancements in surgical methodologies and immunosuppressive treatments, which collectively rendered organ transplantation a feasible endeavor. The landmark accomplishment in this domain occurred in 1954, executed by Dr. Joseph Murray and Dr. David Hume, whose pioneering kidney transplant set the foundation for subsequent advancements. Over successive years, a deeper comprehension of the immune system coupled with the invention of more potent immunosuppressive medications has markedly elevated kidney transplant success rates. Nevertheless, persistent hurdles such as organ rejection and potential complications arising from immune responses continue to pose substantial challenges within the sphere of kidney transplantation research. A thorough grasp of the historical context of kidney transplantation is indispensable for formulating approaches aimed at enhancing outcomes and ensuring the prolonged success of transplant patients [1].

1.2 Role of the complement system

The involvement of the complement system in the setting of kidney transplantation holds significant importance for both innate and adaptive immune responses linked to the phenomenon of allograft rejection. The complement cascade's activation might proceed via the classical, lectin, or alternative pathways, subsequently resulting in the production of anaphylatoxins and opsonins, alongside the formation of the membrane attack complex. This process serves not only to escalate inflammation but also to inflict direct damage upon the endothelium of the allograft, thereby facilitating both acute and chronic rejection. Furthermore, the components of the complement system are being progressively acknowledged as biomarkers for detecting allograft injury, thereby offering valuable insights into the immunological mechanisms that underpin rejection phenomena. Notwithstanding the advancements made in immunosuppressive therapies aimed at curtailing complement activation, further investigative efforts remain necessary to enhance the understanding of the complex interplay between the complement system and immune responses in the context of kidney transplantation. This understanding bears the potential to generate more precisely targeted and efficacious strategies, ultimately contributing to improved transplant outcomes and extended lifespan of graft survival [2].

1.3 Significance of complement activation in kidney transplantation

The significance of complement activation in kidney transplantation is paramount as it is crucial in both the immune response toward the allograft and subsequent outcomes for the recipient. Activation of the complement system causes inflammation, tissue damage, and ultimately rejection of graft. Studies indicate complement activation association with early allograft dysfunction and acute rejection. Mechanisms understanding by which the complement system gets activated in the kidney transplantation context is essential for developing targeted therapies for improving transplant outcomes. Further, research continuing to uncover intricate interactions of complement proteins and various immune cells in allograft rejection emphasizes the immune response complexity in this context. By elucidating the complement activation role, novel therapeutic target identification is potentially possible to enhance graft survival and long-term patient outcomes [3].

2. Overview of complement system

The complement system constitutes a significant element of the innate immune response, performing an essential role in immune surveillance, host defense, and inflammation. Activation of the complement system may occur through three principal pathways: the classical pathway, the lectin pathway, and the alternative pathway. The classical pathway commences through antigen-antibody complexes, whereas the lectin pathway is stimulated by specific sugar motifs on pathogens. Conversely, the alternative pathway is perpetually active at a low level, functioning as a surveillance mechanism. The activation of any of these pathways induces a sequence of enzymatic reactions, which eventually lead to the assembly of membrane attack complexes that lyse target cells. Dysfunction of the complement system has been linked with a variety of pathological conditions, such as autoimmune diseases, inflammatory disorders, and rejection in transplantation. Comprehending the complex mechanisms of complement activation is paramount for developing targeted therapeutic measures in the context of kidney transplantation [4].

2.1 Components of the complement system

The complement setup encompasses a convoluted web of proteins integral to the immune reaction, chiefly in discerning and annihilating pathogens. Activation of the complement system occurs via three principal routes: the classical pathway, the lectin pathway, and the alternative pathway. Each pathway is triggered differently: the classical by antigen-antibody conglomerates, the lectin by mannose-binding lectin, and the alternative by spontaneously hydrolyzed C3 [2]. Post activation, these routes converge at the C3 convertase formation, leading to the cleavage of C3 and subsequent creation of strong effector molecules. These molecules not merely intensify the immune response through the recruitment of inflammatory cells but also engage in opsonization and the direct disintegration of target cells. Grasping the complex elements of the complement system is fundamental for clarifying its involvement in kidney transplants and formulating precise therapeutic strategies.

2.2 Activation pathways

In the realm of kidney transplantation, grasping the pathways responsible for the activation of the complement system proves itself pivotal to overseeing outcomes following transplantation. Activation of the complement system can occur via three principal pathways: the classical pathway, the lectin pathway, and the alternative pathway. Each pathway holds a distinct role in the immune reaction to foreign antigens, which includes the newly transplanted kidney. The classical pathway gets triggered by antigen-antibody complexes, the lectin pathway is initiated through carbohydrate recognition, and the alternative pathway involves spontaneous hydrolysis of C3. Of kidney transplantation, any disturbance within these pathways may result in graft rejection and other related complications. The investigation has demonstrated that specific targeting of elements within these pathways has the potential to adjust the immune response, thereby bettering transplant outcomes. A deep comprehension of the complexities involved in complement activation pathways is indispensable for the advancement of targeted therapeutic approaches that could boost success rates in transplantation [3].

2.3 Regulation of the complement system

The regulation of what is known as the complement system stands as being highly significant in contributing to the maintaining of homeostasis and the prevention of both excessive inflammation and tissue damage. Among the various regulatory proteins, Factor H, Factor I, and membrane-bound regulators perform key functions concerning controlling complement activation upon host cells. To elaborate, Factor H happens to work as a cofactor for Factor I when it comes to the cleavage of C3b, thereby preventing the deposition thereof on self-cells. Furthermore, membrane-bound regulators, specifically those identified as CD55 and CD59, are indispensable to the protection of host cells from complement-mediated lysis. The whole aspect of dysregulation of these regulatory mechanisms can potentially culminate in autoimmune diseases, inflammatory conditions, and tissue injury. As an illustration, within the context of kidney transplantation, upregulation in terms of complement regulatory proteins on donor kidneys proceeds to enhance their resistance to complement-mediated damage, thereby improving graft survival. Comprehending the intricate regulatory pathways of the complement system stands as crucial for the designing and developing of targeted therapies to modulate its activity in distinct disease states. By utilizing this knowledge, researchers can potentially seek to enhance the outcomes of both kidney transplantation and other disorders related to the complement system [3].

3. Immunological basis of kidney transplant rejection

Developments in transplantation sciences have underscored the negative effects of anti-human leukocyte antigen (HLA) antibodies, not only in kidney transplants, but also in heart, lung, and composite tissue transplants. The existence and complement-binding ability of donor-specific anti-HLA antibodies (DSA) are crucial in predicting patient outcomes after transplantation, with those that bind complement being linked to a higher risk of graft failure. Examination of tissue samples shows the damaging impact of DSA on transplanted organs, notably C1q-positive, complement-binding DSA causing increased vascular inflammation and rejection indicators. Incorporating the complement-binding ability of DSA into risk prediction frameworks improves the detection of high-risk patients, promoting personalized treatment plans in solid organ transplants. These observations emphasize the essential role of alloimmune reactions driven by anti-HLA antibodies in kidney transplant rejection and suggest targeted therapies focused on complement control to enhance patient outcomes in transplantation [5]. Contemporary studies also highlight the complex interaction between humoral and cellular immune responses in graft damage and healing, pointing to the potential of new treatments aimed at humoral rejection processes and investigating new strategies for tissue regeneration in transplantation. Recognizing humoral rejection pathways and effectors lays the groundwork for developing targeted anti-humoral therapies, while fresh concepts on tissue regeneration open doors for novel therapeutic solutions to transplantation-related issues [6].

3.1 Types of rejection

Kidney transplantation, though a pivotal solution to ESRD, encounters a persisting challenge in the form of rejection. Innovations in enzymatic blood group conversion have surfaced with the potential to lessen hyperacute antibody-mediated rejection, particularly in ABO-incompatible scenarios [7]. Nonetheless, the intricacy of rejection mechanisms goes past blood group compatibility. Complement activation, acknowledged as a key entity in allograft injury pathways, introduces a numerous difficulty to kidney transplantation [8]. The various rejection forms, such as antibody-mediated rejection and complement-oriented injury, highlight the necessity for personalized therapeutic approaches to better transplant outcomes. The inclusion of new biomarkers for complement activation alongside targeted complement inhibitors in post-transplantation management schemes might pave the way to tackling rejection challenges more effectively and enhancing graft survival rates in kidney transplantation.

3.2 Role of complement activation in rejection

Contemporary investigations have elucidated the pivotal function that complement activation assumes in the rejection of transplanted kidneys. Complement proteins have evidenced themselves as facilitators in the immunological response prompted by the presence of alien antigens inherent to the allograft. Specifically, the induction of the classical and alternative complement pathways incites inflammation and tissue detriment within the transplanted organ. This sequence of phenomena ultimately converges in the aggregation of immune cells and the obliteration of the donor tissue. Empirical inquiries have indicated that the inhibition of complement components can substantially mitigate the frequency and severity of rejection incidences, accentuating the significance of this pathway in the rejection continuum. Comprehending the intricacies of complement activation in rejection is imperative for devising targeted therapeutics to ameliorate the prolonged outcomes of kidney transplant recipients [3].

3.3 Impact on graft survival

Additionally, the inquiry into complement activation's effect on graft endurance in kidney transplantation has been a matter of thorough exploration. Research has indicated the activation of the complement system as significant in the development of allograft rejection, influencing outcomes post-transplantation over an extended period. Notably, C4d deposition, indicative of complement activation, correlates with diminished graft survival rates. Furthermore, donor-specific antibodies (DSA) can cause complement-mediated damage to the allograft, leading to acute and chronic rejection [9]. Consequently, strategies targeting the complement system have surfaced as potential therapeutic interventions to bolster graft survival in kidney transplant patients. By delving into the complex mechanisms of complement activation and its effect on transplant results, scientists can formulate novel therapies aimed at improving graft survival and long-term patient health.

4. Complement activation in kidney transplantation

Evidence emerging indicates complement activation's significant involvement in kidney transplant rejection pathogenesis. The presence of complement components in the allograft instigates inflammatory responses which result in tissue damage and graft loss ultimately. Furthermore, complement system dysregulation correlates with antibody-mediated rejection development, recognized as a principal cause of allograft failure. Research indicates targeting specific complement cascade components—like C5 or C3—can reduce inflammation and increase allograft survival rates. Therefore, delving into mechanisms behind complement activation in kidney transplantation is essential for crafting therapeutic strategies aimed at rejection prevention and improvement of allograft outcomes. More research is mandatory to uncover the complex relationship between the complement system and allograft immune responses, which could lead to innovative treatment methods in transplantation medicine [2].

4.1 Mechanisms of complement activation

Additionally, comprehending the mechanisms of complement activation regarding kidney transplantation holds significance for ameliorating clinical outcomes. The complement system can initiate through three principal pathways: the classical pathway, the lectin pathway, and the alternative pathway. In kidney transplantation, the classical pathway is predominantly activated by antibodies binding to antigens on the transplanted organ, culminating in the formation of antigen-antibody complexes. This sequence activates C1q, C4, and C3, thereby leading to the production of anaphylatoxins and opsonins, which may provoke inflammation and tissue damage. In contrast, the lectin pathway is activated by mannose-binding lectin (MBL) attaching to carbohydrate structures on the surface of pathogens or injured cells, whereas the alternative pathway spontaneously activates through a method known as tick-over [2]. By parsing out the specific pathways engaged in complement activation within the context of kidney transplantation, new therapeutic approaches could be formulated to interfere with these mechanisms to avert graft rejection.

4.2 Local versus systemic activation

Recent investigations have underscored the significance of recognizing the differentiation between local and systemic complement activation regarding kidney transplantation. The term local activation pertains to the complement system's activation within the renal allograft itself, resulting in direct tissue damage and inflammation. Conversely, systemic activation denotes the complement cascade's activation within the bloodstream, which might ultimately cause systemic complications like thrombotic microangiopathy. It is imperative to distinguish the respective contributions of local versus systemic complement activation to formulate targeted therapeutic strategies that can specifically tackle the underlying pathophysiological mechanisms. Whereas local complement activation within the allograft could be a primary cause of acute rejection, systemic complement activation might influence the long-term function of the allograft and patient outcomes. Additional research is necessary to clarify the complex interplay between these dual modalities of complement activation in the context of kidney transplantation [2].

4.3 Timing of activation post-transplant

The timing concerning complement activation following transplantation has significant importance in determining the outcomes associated with kidney allografts. Complement activation is deeply involved in IgA nephropathy (IgAN), highlighting the importance of the temporal aspect concerning the activation of the complement pathway in post-transplant situations [10]. Specifically, C4d staining, which is a recognized marker of complement activation, has shown its value in several glomerular diseases, such as in cases of kidney allograft rejection [11]. The capability to recognize C4d through immunohistochemistry on formalin-fixed samples presents a useful approach for evaluating complement activation post-transplant and provides insights into the possible consequences for allograft outcomes. Thus, incorporating a sophisticated understanding of the timing and patterns concerning complement activation post-transplantation, as informed by information from IgAN pathology and complementary methodologies like C4d immunohistochemistry, is crucial for the progression of renal histopathology in the context of kidney transplantation studies.

5. Diagnostic tools for complement activation

The creation of diagnostic tools for the activation of the complement within the framework of kidney transplantation is indispensable for early identification and intervention. Diverse assays have been employed for the quantification of complement activation entities, such as C3a, C4d, and the membrane attack complex (MAC). These assays may offer consequential perceptions of the degree of complement activation and assist in treatment resolutions. Moreover, contemporary methods like flow cytometry and gene expression profiling have displayed the potential role of complement in allograft rejection [2]. The incorporation of these diagnostic apparatuses into standard monitoring protocols might enhance patient prognoses by granting clinicians the ability to detect rejection episodes sooner and modify immunosuppressive strategies correspondingly.

5.1 Laboratory tests

To evaluate complement activation in the context of kidney transplantation, numerous lab tests are usable. These tests are vital in tracking the immune response and identifying potential post-transplant complications. Biomarkers, including levels of C3 and C4 and measurements of complement fragments like C3d and Bb, can yield critical insights into complement system activation and its effects on graft endurance. Additionally, tests that assess the presence of anti-HLA antibodies and complement protein deposits on graft tissue can provide further data regarding the recipient's immunological condition and rejection risks [2]. By integrating these lab tests with clinical information, healthcare practitioners can more precisely tailor immunosuppressive therapies and enhance outcomes for kidney transplant patients.

5.2 Imaging techniques

Imaging methodologies hold pivotal relevance in the scrutinization of complement activation within kidney transplantation. The discernment of complement proteins properdin and C5b-9 in urinary specimens demonstrates a significant correlation with post-transplantation renal failure [37]. This emphasizes the criticality of non-invasive imaging modalities for the identification of complement activation indicators. Furthermore, Stacks [12] accentuate the employment of immunohistochemistry and immunofluorescence in the examination of immunoproteasome and complement system activation in transplanted kidneys subjected to cold preservation. Such imaging strategies contribute not only to the comprehension of renal damage mechanisms but also offer perspectives regarding potential targeted interventions. Through the amalgamation of progressive imaging technologies with complement activation studies, a thorough grasp of the pathophysiology underlying kidney transplant rejection is attainable, ultimately informing the creation of customized therapeutic protocols to enhance patient prognoses.

5.3 Biomarkers

The scrutiny of complement activation within the realm of kidney transplantation emerges as an intricate endeavor, especially concerning IgA nephropathy (IgAN). Scholarly examination of biomarkers, encompassing C3a, C5a, and Bb, has elucidated the nuanced dynamics governing complement regulation in IgAN patients, pivotal for comprehending disease mechanisms and steering therapeutic strategies. The thorough examination of complement activation and regulatory segments, as pinpointed in the examination by Duval et al. [13], discerned distinct groups of patients exhibiting differing complement activity patterns, accentuating the potential merit of precise complement therapies in particular patient subsets. Additionally, the inclusion of serum C3 and C4 values in predictive frameworks has indicated encouraging outcomes in boosting prognostic precision and identifying patients at elevated risk for disease aggravation [14]. These observations highlight the essential influence of biomarkers in refining risk categorization and individualized therapy approaches within the intricate domain of complement-associated kidney ailments such as IgAN.

6. Clinical manifestations of complement activation

The intricate interaction of complement activation in atypical hemolytic uremic syndrome (aHUS) indicates various clinical presentations emerging from the unchecked alternative complement pathway activation. Concerning kidney transplantation, grasping the triad of hemolytic anemia, thrombocytopenia, and acute kidney injury is pivotal for thorough patient management. Moreover, infectious causes like Shiga toxin-producing *Escherichia coli* (STEC) and secondary factors such as cancer or autoimmune disorders can trigger a series of events culminating in renal dysfunction and thrombotic microangiopathy. Eculizumab, a monoclonal antibody that targets the complement C5 protein, has become an essential therapeutic choice, providing significant remission rates and recovery of renal function in aHUS patients. Nonetheless, careful consideration should be given to the ideal duration of eculizumab treatment to avert relapses, particularly in patients with identified risk factors like rare complement gene variants or heightened soluble C5b-9 levels after discontinuation [15, 16].

6.1 Acute rejection

To delve into the scrutiny of acute rejection within the context of kidney transplantation mandates a thorough grasp of intricate processes attributive to immune-mediated allograft damage. Prevailing investigative endeavors have elucidated the import of complement activation in the context of antibody-mediated rejection (ABMR) along with its conceivable diagnostic pertinence. There exists research probing markers indicative of complement activation, encompassing C3, C3d, C5b-9, and

C4d, within systemic and intrarenal realms, aimed at differentiating rejection types. Of particular note, C3d deposition has surfaced as a distinctly discriminative element in the diagnostic sphere of active ABMR, specifically within glomerular and peritubular capillaries. Furthermore, the scrutiny of urinary markers such as sVCAM-1 and sC4d has shown prospective utility in discerning between rejection episodes, positing their potential as non-invasive diagnostic instruments. Collectively, these findings accentuate the pivotal role of grasping and overseeing complement activation within acute rejection contexts, thereby enriching patient management and outcomes in kidney transplantation scenarios.

6.2 Chronic allograft dysfunction

Grasping the molecular and cellular mechanisms that are fundamental to chronic allograft dysfunction in kidney transplantation is critical for upgrading results in transplant patients. The employment of advanced technologies, for instance, digital spatial profiling (DSP) and comprehensive transcriptome analysis, bestows significant revelations into the specific cell types and molecular routes implicated in allograft failure, as shown in Dorr et al. [17]. Recognizing key agents like macrophages and singling out transcriptomic markers related to graft outcomes, researchers might unveil novel therapeutic targets to bolster immune suppression tactics. Furthermore, the import of the complement system in allograft injury, emphasized in Golshayan et al. [8], accentuates the importance of assessing complement activation in post-transplant management to reduce kidney damage. Specific interventions aimed at complement pathways might prove beneficial in averting chronic antibody-mediated rejection and boosting long-term transplant success.

6.3 Antibody-mediated rejection

The issue of antibody-mediated rejection (AMR) persists as a formidable obstacle in the domain of kidney transplantation, presenting a hazard to graft viability. In instances of AMR, preformed antibodies or newly formed donor-specific antibodies attack the allograft, which incites complement activation, endothelial damage, and, eventually, graft malfunction. The classical complement pathway's activation is pivotal in AMR development, fostering tissue harm and inflammatory processes. Furthermore, complement activation derivatives like C3a and C5a can attract inflammatory cells and intensify the immune reaction against the allograft. Strategies that aim at complement system inhibition indicate potential in diminishing AMR and improving transplantation results, underlining the therapeutic promise of targeting complement mechanisms in kidney transplants [18]. There is a need for further investigatory efforts to comprehend the detailed interactions between antibodies, complement activation, and allograft damage in AMR.

7. Therapeutic approaches targeting complement system

Therapeutic methodologies aiming at the complement system within renal transplantation have manifested potential outcomes in enhancing graft performance. One method incorporates the employment of complement inhibitors to obstruct the initiation of the complement cascade, which holds a crucial part in the development of both acute and chronic rejection. Specifically, addressing particular elements of the complement framework, such as C5 or C3, has demonstrated efficacy in diminishing the inflammatory reaction linked with allograft rejection. Additionally, therapy focusing on the complement has the prospective benefit of decreasing the occurrence of antibody-mediated rejection, a significant contributor to graft failure in renal transplantation [4]. These revelations highlight the necessity of forging innovative therapeutic techniques that attentively target the complement system to support long-term transplantation results.

7.1 Pharmacological inhibition

The issue of complement activation significantly challenges renal transplantation, necessitating a detailed strategy for pharmacological suppression. As mentioned by Bernuy-Guevara et al. [19], the terminal complement component 5 (C5) blockers such as eculizumab and ravulizumab show effectiveness in reducing hemolysis in paroxysmal nocturnal hemoglobinuria and in controlling thrombotic microangiopathy in atypical hemolytic uremic syndrome, highlighting their potential in lessening post-transplantation complications. Additionally, Lammerts [37] highlight the involvement of complement activation in antibody-mediated rejection following transplantation, explaining molecular mechanisms and the potential for personalized immunosuppressive methods. By synthesizing insights from these researches, one gains a nuanced perception of the effects of complement inhibitors on kidney allograft results, underlining the necessity for specific treatment schemes to tackle complement-related obstacles in kidney transplant recipients.

7.2 Complement blockade

When one contemplates the importance of the activation of complement in the context of kidney transplants, particularly relating to antibody-mediated rejection (AMR), the consideration of complement blockade becomes essential for therapeutic intervention. As elaborated upon by Thomas et al. [20], the preventive effects of monoclonal antibodies aimed at C1s against HLA antibody-provoked complement deposition highlight the possibility of using specific complement modulation to lessen the harmful consequences of donor-specific antibodies on endothelial cells. Additionally, as detailed in Noris and Remuzzi [21], improper complement activation presents a severe threat for inflammatory damage in the kidneys, connecting complement dysregulation to several renal conditions. By utilizing strategies of complement blockade, such as TNT003, there arises the hopeful outlook of reducing complement-related damage within the context of kidney transplants, thereby reducing the chances of negative results caused by overactive inflammatory responses.

7.3 Novel therapies

In the domain of kidney transplantation, there is an emerging interest in exploring new therapies aimed at enhancing outcomes and reducing complications linked to the procedure. These therapies include a diverse array of approaches, spanning from novel pharmacological agents to advanced surgical methods. By focusing on critical pathways in complement activation, such as the lectin pathway, these innovative therapies possess significant potential for decreasing rejection rates and improving graft survival. For instance, recent research has indicated the effectiveness of new complement inhibitors in averting complement-mediated harm in renal allografts.

Moreover, advanced immunomodulatory approaches, like personalized immunosuppressive regimens tailored to the specific profiles of patients, are increasingly being utilized to enhance post-transplant outcomes. Looking ahead, additional studies are necessary to assess the long-term efficacy and safety of these new therapies within the kidney transplantation context.

8. Impact of complement activation on patient outcomes

Hence, the significance of comprehending the ramifications of complement activation concerning patient outcomes within kidney transplantation cannot be overstated. The activation of the complement system is capable of engendering varied pathophysiological responses, including but not limited to inflammation, tissue damage, and the modulation of immune response. Such processes hold considerable relevance to the success of kidney transplantation and the patient's overall health status. Empirical evidence has indicated that an excessive or dysregulated activation of the complement system may substantively contribute to allograft rejection, delayed graft function, and potential graft loss. Through the elucidation of mechanisms by which complement activation influences patient outcomes in the realm of kidney transplantation, healthcare professionals can pinpoint novel therapeutic targets, thereby enhancing transplant success rates and prolonging patient survival. Consequently, additional investigation in this domain is pivotal for augmenting our grasp of the complex interactions between the complement system and patient outcomes within kidney transplantation.

8.1 Graft survival rates

The intricate interplay existing between complement activation and the post-transplant outcomes of kidney transplantation has critical implications for graft survival rates. The recurrence of rare conditions such as C3 glomerulopathy represents a notable threat to recipients, with over 50% encountering recurrence after transplant, thus extensively contributing to graft loss after rejection [22]. To address these associated risks, the investigation into anti-complement therapies like eculizumab and ravalizumab has revealed optimistic results in managing C3 glomerulopathy among transplant patients. Furthermore, the complex dynamics of ischemia-reperfusion injury impacting proximal tubular epithelial cells highlight the necessity of comprehending complement regulatory proteins, such as CD59, in hypoxia and reoxygenation scenarios, which have implications for C3 deposition and, consequently, graft outcomes [23]. Conducting a thorough assessment of complement activation in the realm of kidney transplantation is essential for enhancing graft survival rates and progressing transplant care.

8.2 Patient morbidity

Individuals subjected to kidney transplantation encounter substantial morbidity risks, where ailments such as chronic kidney disease (CKD) and acute kidney injury (AKI) present elevated mortality threats. The exclusion criteria of patients with preestablished CKD from hematopoietic stem cell transplantation (HSCT) underscore the vital role of renal functionality in transplant prognoses. Research inspecting kidney injury biomarkers in HSCT patients reveals heightened IGFBP-7/TIMP2, netrin-1, and semaphorin A2 levels, suggesting possible kidney impairment even among those manifesting ostensibly normal post-transplant renal function. Concurrently, patients undergoing hemodialysis suffer from numerous complications, including immune system dysregulation encompassing both innate and adaptive responses, resulting in persistent inflammation and increased morbidity. Tackling immune dysfunction in these patients could pave the way for better outcomes and diminished mortality risks, underscoring the essential demand for nephroprotective measures and immune system interventions in susceptible cohorts undergoing transplantations or hemodialysis [24, 25].

8.3 Long-term complications

The intricacies involved in kidney transplantation are not limited to the immediate period after surgery, as enduring complications significantly influence patient outcomes. Although research like [26] has focused on the effects of surgical timing on both patient and graft survival, further investigation is crucial to comprehend the factors that contribute to long-term complications. Complement activation, highlighted in Moldakhmetova et al. [23], especially when considering ischemia-reperfusion injury, stands out as a pivotal mechanism that impacts the success of kidney transplants. The complex relationship between hypoxia, reoxygenation, and the modulation of complement components illustrates the delicate equilibrium needed for maintaining optimal graft functionality over an extended period. By delving into the molecular intricacies of complement activation within renal epithelial cells, we can develop targeted strategies to alleviate long-term complications and enhance graft longevity, opening new possibilities for improving transplantation outcomes.

9. Complement system and ischemia-reperfusion injury

The intricate interplay between elements of the complement system and ischemia-reperfusion injury during kidney transplantation presents a highly complex phenomenon necessitating thorough investigation. Gaining an understanding of the dysregulation of primary complement components like C3 and C5, along with their activation fragments and specific receptors, proves critical in deciphering the pathophysiology associated with renal damage post-transplantation. Utilizing antioxidant polypropylene sulfide nanoparticles (PPS-NPs) in processes such as cold storage and normothermic machine perfusion (NMP) appears to offer a strategy worth considering for mitigating oxidative stress and inflammation characteristic of ischemia-reperfusion injury. By scavenging reactive oxygen species and curtailing complement activation, PPS-NPs apparently enhance organ viability and function meaningfully, thereby potentially expanding the donor kidney pool. Additionally, delving into the dysregulation of the complement system in diverse kidney disorders underscores its critical role within renal pathology, warranting further investigation to fully understand its ramifications in conditions including renal cell carcinoma and various other malignancies.

9.1 Pathophysiology

Additionally, comprehending the pathophysiology linked to complement activation holds indispensable significance in the purview of kidney transplantation. The intricate interactions existing between innate and adaptive immune systems that implicate several complement components are capable of imparting notable impacts on allograft results. Activation of the complement system might take place via classical, lectin, or alternative pathways, culminating in inflammation, tissue injury, and eventuating in allograft rejection. For instance, ischemia-reperfusion injury experienced during the transplantation procedure might incite complement cascades, aggravating renal tissue damage and impinging on graft functionality. Moreover, persistent antibody-mediated rejection typified by the emergence of donor-specific antibodies and ensuing complement activation stands as a formidable obstacle to the prolonged survival of the allograft. Hence, acquiring a deeper insight into the pathophysiological mechanisms governing complement activation in the context of kidney transplantation is imperative for formulating precise therapeutic strategies aimed at enhancing transplant results [2].

9.2 Role in acute injury

In the context of kidney transplants, a matter necessitating in-depth analysis concerns the role of complement activation in acute injury phases. Research illustrated in Yerly et al. [27] highlights the possible importance of halting terminal complement cascade, notably using eculizumab to reduce acute antibody-mediated rejection (AMR) in heart transplant patients. Additionally, the investigation noted by Castellano et al. [28] points out the role of complement in triggering pericyte-to-myofibroblast transdifferentiation (PMT) after renal ischemia/reperfusion injury, stressing the effects on microvascular stability. These findings underline the complex interaction between complement activation and acute injury mechanisms in kidney transplants, indicating potential targeted therapies like C1-INH. A deeper grasp of complement-driven tissue damage could foster progress in developing strategies to lessen acute injury reactions post-transplantation.

9.3 Therapeutic interventions

Moreover, the interventions with therapeutic goals aimed at adjusting complement activation in kidney transplantation have indicated promising outcomes. One approach to consider encompasses the employment of complement inhibitors to specifically target components within the complement cascade. For instance, utilization of C5 inhibitors has been demonstrated to notably decrease complement-mediated damage in renal allografts. Additionally, strategies that concentrate on targeting complement receptors or regulatory elements have surfaced as potential therapeutic options. By adjusting these crucial components of the complement system, researchers remain hopeful in attenuating the harmful impacts of complement activation on allograft survival [2]. These innovative therapeutic interventions are not only very promising for enhancing outcomes in kidney transplantation, but they also symbolize a novel pathway for research within the domain of immunology and transplantation medicine.

10. Complement system and donor-specific antibodies

The existence of donor-specific antibodies (DSAs) in the context of kidney transplantation introduces a substantial difficulty due to the link with graft rejection and unfavorable results. Research has indicated that the complement system holds a pivotal role in the DSAs' activation, culminating in antibody-mediated rejection (AMR). When DSAs bind to donor antigens, activation of the classical complement pathway occurs, which leads to the creation of the membrane attack complex and ensuing tissue harm. Moreover, complement fragment deposition on endothelial cells can escalate inflammation and thrombosis, worsening the rejection scenario. Grasping the relationship between the complement system and DSAs is vital for crafting targeted therapies aimed at preventing and controlling AMR in kidney transplants. Continued investigation in this domain is necessary to identify potential therapeutic targets and enhance outcomes for transplant recipients [29].

10.1 Relationship with antibody-mediated rejection

The complex interaction between complement activation and antibody-mediated rejection (AMR) in kidney transplantation proposes a convoluted pathophysiological enigma. Research has accentuated the import of Factor H-related proteins (FHRs) in modulating complement activation within allografts, especially under inflammatory circumstances. Remarkably, FHR-3 deposition has been observed in kidney allografts, mainly confined to podocytes, in both rejection and non-rejection scenarios. This observation highlights FHRs' potential role in complement dysregulation amidst post-transplant inflammatory responses. Furthermore, in ABO-incompatible kidney transplantation, persistent complement activation by anti-ABO antibodies has been linked with T-cell-mediated rejection and compromised long-term graft function. The correlation between pre-transplant anti-ABO antibody titers, complement activation indicators, and rejection incidents elucidates the intricate association between antibody-mediated processes, complement components, and graft outcomes in kidney transplantation. Collectively, these findings pinpoint the multifarious nature of complement-related pathways in the context of AMR, accentuating the necessity for further clarification of these complex interactions to ameliorate therapeutic approaches and enhance transplant results.

10.2 Influence on graft survival

Multiple determinants exert considerable effects on graft endurance post-kidney transplantation. Noteworthy among these is the complement system's activation, integral to the immune reaction against the transplanted organ. The activation cascade of the complement system culminates in inflammation, inflicting tissue damage, and eventually, graft rejection. Empirical evidence has demonstrated a correlation between heightened levels of complement activation derivatives, such as C3a and C5a, and unfavorable graft prognoses. Furthermore, genetic polymorphisms within complement-related genes correlate with a heightened susceptibility to acute rejection and diminished graft longevity [29]. Analyzing the ramifications of complement activation on graft viability is pivotal for formulating targeted immunosuppressive protocols aimed at augmenting long-term transplant success. Through dissecting the mechanisms driving complement-induced graft damage, ensuing research endeavors might pinpoint innovative therapeutic avenues to bolster graft durability and enhance patient prognoses.

10.3 Treatment considerations

Given the intricate nature of complement activation in kidney transplantation, clinicians must evaluate various therapeutic strategies. Primarily, therapies focusing on specific complement components, such as eculizumab, indicate potential in averting complement-mediated renal damage. Additionally, approaches aimed at regulating the entire complement system, including complement inhibitors or blocking complement receptors, could provide innovative methods to alleviate the adverse effects of complement activation within the transplantation context [30]. Moreover, individualized treatment strategies, customized to the complement profile and risk elements of particular patients, might be crucial to enhancing outcomes in kidney transplant recipients. Through meticulous consideration of these treatment aspects, healthcare professionals can potentially improve the success rates of kidney transplantation while mitigating the risks linked with complement activation.

11. Complement system and HLA mismatch

In the realm of kidney transplantation, the involvement of the complement system and HLA mismatch significantly influences graft results. The human leukocyte antigens (HLA) are crucial in defining immune reactions, with mismatched HLA being primary targets for the immune mechanism. Pre-existing donor-specific HLA antibodies notably can result in antibody-mediated rejection, a major reason for early allograft failures post-transplant [31]. It is important to grasp how HLA antibodies trigger the complement system and cause endothelial harm for forecasting and controlling graft outcomes. Additionally, the existence of neutralizing antibodies, such as those detected against BK polyomavirus in immunoglobulin formulations, highlights the possible therapeutic approaches aimed at specific complement pathways, showing the complex link between the complement system and immune reactions in kidney transplant contexts. This active interaction indicates the necessity for thorough evaluations and tailored interventions to enhance transplant success amid the complicated interplay of immune factors.

11.1 Association with rejection

Recent investigatory outputs have illuminated an influential presence of complement-fixing de novo donor-specific antibodies (dnDSA) on the processes of rejection and the results of renal graft among recipients of kidney transplants [32]. These discoveries underscore the essential participation of complement activation in post-transplantation antibody-mediated rejection (AMR). Further studies focusing on donor C3 allotypes' impact on renal transplant consequences have disclosed noteworthy observations [33]. Explicitly, a donor's C3 (F) allele existence, whether in homozygous or heterozygous forms, combined with its absence in recipients, correlates with better renal allograft performance. Comprehending the intricate interactions between complement-fixing antibodies and specific genetic factors of donors is pivotal for personalizing treatment regimens and predicting AMR consequences. Applying these insights in clinical settings might improve risk assessment and long-term graft survival efficacy for kidney transplant recipients.

11.2 Impact on transplant outcomes

Further, the repercussions of complement activation on transplant outcomes should not be overlooked. The activation of the complement system in kidney transplantation scenarios has been connected to an elevated risk of early graft dysfunction, acute rejection episodes, as well as diminished survival rates of the allograft on a long-term basis.

The accumulation of complement proteins within the transplanted kidney can instigate localized inflammation and tissue injury, thereby contributing to adverse outcomes following transplantation. Complement activation has also been linked to antibody-mediated rejection development, an acute complication which endangers graft function significantly. Gaining an understanding of the complement's role in transplant results is paramount for the creation of targeted therapeutic strategies aimed at enhancing graft survival rates. By uncovering the underlying mechanisms by which complement activation affects transplant outcomes, both clinicians and researchers might pinpoint novel tactics to support the success rates of kidney transplantation [34].

11.3 Strategies for HLA matching

In the realm of kidney transplantation, significant attention is paid to the harmonization of the human leukocyte antigen (HLA) between the donor and recipient as a means to curtail the risk of rejection. A multitude of methodologies have been conceived to refine HLA matching and advance transplant results. One method involves concentrating on the matching of HLA-A, HLA-B, and HLA-DR antigens, given that such matching is correlated with enhanced graft survival rates. Another tactic encompasses virtual crossmatching, entailing the use of algorithms to surmise the probability of compatibility predicated on HLA typing outcomes [30]. Moreover, the employment of desensitization protocols might be beneficial in surmounting immunological impediments in highly sensitized patients by mitigating antibody levels and expanding the spectrum of feasible donors. Through the adoption of these assorted methodologies for HLA matching, transplant centers potentially amplify the efficaciousness of kidney transplantation and augment patient prognoses.

12. Complement system and endothelial activation

The complex relationship between the complement system and endothelial activation is of major importance within kidney transplantation. Research has highlighted the essential role of complement inhibition in reducing ischemia-reperfusion injury (IRI) and antibody-mediated rejection (ABMR) after transplantation. Significantly, the application of C1 inhibitor (C1-INH) stands out as a potentially effective therapeutic method, as it targets the early stages of complement activation and also affects non-complement pathways and interactions between leukocytes and endothelial cells [35]. This layered approach could likely improve graft results by decreasing IRI and improving delayed graft function, particularly in high-risk grafts. Furthermore, the wider consequences of complement dysregulation on endothelial dysfunction emphasize the necessity for thorough strategies that address both proximal and distal complement pathways, as discussed in the developing field of complement therapeutics [36]. These observations emphasize the complex dynamics of complement activation in kidney transplantation, underlining the importance of specific interventions to improve graft survival and performance.

12.1 Endothelial cell damage

Damage to endothelial cells exhibits significant relevance in the pathogenesis of allograft rejection following kidney transplantation. An important contributor to such endothelial damage is the activation of the complement cascade, which results in endothelial dysfunction and eventual organ damage. Components of the complement system, specifically C3a and C5a, have been identified as mediators in the activation of endothelial cells and in the recruitment of inflammatory cells to the sites of injury. This process further intensifies the immune response and enhances tissue damage within the allograft. Moreover, activation of the complement system can result in the creation of membrane attack complexes, which cause direct lysis of endothelial cells and compromise the integrity of the vascular endothelium [2]. Addressing the complement system can potentially offer a therapeutic solution to lessen endothelial cell damage and improve long-term outcomes in individuals receiving kidney transplants.

12.2 Vascular complications

The complex interplay regarding complement activation coupled with vascular complications in the context of kidney transplantation illuminates a multifaceted scenario warranting detailed examination. As presented by Lammerts [37], finding complement proteins properdine and C5b-9 in urine after transplantation is strongly linked to kidney failure, highlighting the key role complement plays in outcomes related to grafts. Additionally, Nieuwenhuijs-Moeke et al. [35] explores approaches such as pharmacological conditioning and ischemic conditioning at a distance aimed at reducing injury post-surgery and enhancing graft functionality. Nevertheless, the effectiveness of such methods remains debated. Comprehending how complement activation relates to vascular complications following transplantation is critical to improving results for patients and refining therapeutic techniques. By examining how dysregulation of the complement cascade impacts vascular integrity, new perspectives might be gained to guide specialized interventions addressing vascular issues in recipients of kidney transplants, thus potentially influencing the course of postoperative results.

12.3 Endothelial protection strategies

Recent progressions in discerning the molecular circuits implicated in ischemia-reperfusion injury (IRI) after kidney transplantation have illuminated feasible paths for augmenting graft endurance. The intricate pathological occurrence of IRI, as detailed in Nieuwenhuijs-Moeke et al. [35], accentuates the imperative of formulating specific therapeutic tactics to attenuate its adverse impacts. Notably, the engagement of complement activation in renal failure post-transplantation, as revealed in Lammerts [37], underscores the complex interaction between the immune system and transplanted organs. Such revelations elucidate the critical need to scrutinize endothelial safeguarding strategies as a method to boost graft functionality and mitigate rejection probabilities. By probing the fundamentals of complement activation and its ramifications for transplant outcomes, scholars can enhance methodologies geared toward sustaining endothelial cohesion and elevating transplant achievements. Embedding these discoveries into all-encompassing treatment schemas might foster ground-breaking therapies that tackle the multifaceted interface between the complement mechanism and graft viability in kidney transplants.

13. Complement system and fibrosis

Moreover, in fibrotic disease pathogenesis, dysregulation of the complement system is implicated, inclusive of renal fibrosis being an instance. Complement system activation can consequently lead to pro-inflammatory cytokines generation, immune cell recruitment, and extracellular matrix protein production, cumulatively contributing to tissue fibrosis. Pertinent to kidney transplantation, complement activation can be precipitated by ischemia-reperfusion injury and acute rejection, potentially promoting the development of interstitial fibrosis and tubular atrophy [38]. Comprehending the complicated interplay between the complement system and fibrosis within the realm of renal transplantation holds significance for formulating targeted therapies aimed at either preventing or mitigating fibrotic transformations in transplanted kidneys. By clarifying the mechanisms behind complement-mediated fibrosis, innovative treatment strategies could be conceived, making long-term outcomes in transplantation recipients realistic.

13.1 Fibrotic processes

The interaction between the activation of complement and fibrotic processes within kidney transplantation produces numerous complexities that notably influence graft outcomes. Fibrosis, which is typified by the excessive accumulation of extracellular matrix proteins like collagen, emerges as a significant factor in chronic graft dysfunction. Activation of complement is evidenced to directly drive fibrotic responses by way of attracting immune cells and facilitating the release of pro-inflammatory cytokines. Additionally, complement activation can strengthen fibrosis through the activation of endothelial cells and the remodeling of tissue. Research has indicated that inhibition of certain complement components holds the potential to lessen fibrotic processes in various disease contexts, pointing toward a potential therapeutic focus for impeding fibrosis in renal allografts. Grasping the nuanced interplay between complement activation and fibrosis proves critical for formulating targeted strategies aimed at enhancing the long-term survival of grafts [39].

13.2 Impact on allograft fibrosis

Within allografts, the existing stromal vascular fraction has evidenced potential in attenuating acute renal ischemia/reperfusion injury along with fibrosis, highlighting the capability for therapeutic measures aimed at enhancing allograft results [40]. Conversely, the activation of complement, particularly via C4d accretion in peritubular capillaries, has demonstrated a correlation with antibody-mediated rejection in renal allografts, bearing significant consequences for graft viability. Research has pinpointed a marked link between C4d presence and negative outcomes such as graft failure, even when rejection instances are not observed. These results emphasize the pivotal influence of complement activation on allograft fibrosis and overall renal performance. The intricate relationship among immune reactions, complement activation, and allograft fibrosis illustrates the intricateness of renal transplant dynamics and underscores the necessity for precise therapeutic approaches to foster improved long-term graft prognoses.

13.3 Antifibrotic therapies

Fibrosis constitutes a frequently observed pathological development within kidney transplantation scenarios, potentially resulting in dysfunction and ultimate failure of grafts. A promising avenue to address this issue involves antifibrotic therapies, which engage varied pathways implicated in fibrosis pathogenesis, including but not limited to TGF-β signaling, inflammatory mechanisms, and oxidative stress effects. For instance, the antifibrotic compound pirfenidone, which has received approval for therapeutic use in idiopathic pulmonary fibrosis, has manifested encouraging outcomes in preclinical investigations regarding renal fibrosis. Furthermore, angiotensin-converting enzyme inhibitors and angiotensin receptor blockers, drugs traditionally utilized in the management of hypertension, have also displayed antifibrotic capacities within kidney disease contexts. However, despite the progress marked by such advances, additional research remains imperative to enhance the application of antifibrotic therapies within kidney transplant procedures and to advance long-term prognoses for transplant recipients [41].

14. Conclusion

The complex interaction between complement activation and kidney transplant results highlights the need for more research in this domain. Even with advancements in acknowledging complement's role in organ rejection, notable knowledge gaps still exist. Forthcoming investigations should focus on clarifying the precise methods through which complement activation leads to kidney damage after transplantation and recognize potential therapeutic targets to reduce its harmful impacts. Furthermore, clinical trials are required to assess the effectiveness and safety of therapies aimed at complementing in stopping organ rejection and boosting long-term graft viability. By broadening our comprehension of immune reactions mediated by complement in kidney transplants, it is possible to improve patient outcomes and lessen the chronic issues associated with allograft function.

14.1 Implications for clinical practice

Moreover, the ramifications for clinical praxis within the scope of complement activation amid kidney transplantation are considerable. Comprehending complement's influence on allograft repudiation and harm can precipitate the creation of pinpoint therapeutic measures to ameliorate patient prognoses. For example, complement inhibitors such as eculizumab hold the potential to hinder antibody-mediated rejection among kidney transplant recipients. By integrating complement inhibition into conventional immunosuppressive protocols, practitioners might diminish the peril of acute and chronic allograft damage. Moreover, pinpointing biomarkers denoting complement activation in kidney transplant patients may facilitate the preliminary detection of rejection episodes, permitting swift intervention and possibly supporting graft survival rates. In sum, the incorporation of complement-focused therapies within clinical practice promises the potential to transform the management of kidney transplantation and elevate patient outcomes.

14.2 Future research directions

Incremental developments within the sphere of preclinical xenotransplant investigations have brought to prominence possible clinical ramifications related to renal transplantation by underscoring the essentiality of genetic alterations in porcine donors. Probing has unveiled that the nullification of the CMAH gene within pigs leads to a reduction in antibody-mediated inflammatory and coagulative responses, thereby augmenting human transplant compatibility [42]. The comprehension of complement activation's role in renal pathologies proves pivotal for enhancing transplantation outcomes. The importance of urinary complement biomarkers as non-invasive markers of renal inflammation reveals a promising direction for subsequent inquiries. Through continued explorations and validations related to urinary complement biomarkers in evaluating disease activity, forecasting therapeutic responses, and directing intervention strategies, researchers are poised to ameliorate the management of complement-mediated renal injuries in transplant scenarios [43]. Attempts to delineate complement activation mechanisms alongside devising dependable biomarkers possess substantial promise for the progression of the renal transplantation area.

Author details

Pande Made Wisnu Tirtayasa[1*], Gerhard Reinaldi Situmorang[2], Gede Wirya Kusuma Duarsa[3], Arry Rodjani[2] and Nur Rasyid[2]

1 Faculty of Medicine Universitas Udayana, Department of Urology, Universitas Udayana Teaching Hospital, Bali, Indonesia

2 Faculty of Medicine Universitas Indonesia, Department of Urology, Cipto Mangunkusumo National Referral Hospital, Jakarta, Indonesia

3 Faculty of Medicine Universitas Udayana, Department of Urology, Prof. dr. I.G.N.G. Ngoerah General Hospital, Bali, Indonesia

*Address all correspondence to: wisnu.tirtayasa@gmail.com

References

[1] Van Zanden JE, Jager NM, Daha MR, Erasmus ME, Leuvenink HGD, Seelen MA. Complement therapeutics in the multi-organ donor: Do or don't? Frontiers in Immunology. 2019;**10**:329. DOI: 10.3389/fimmu.2019.00329

[2] Zipfel PF, editor. Complement and Kidney Disease. Basel, Switzerland: Springer Science; 2006

[3] Pontrelli P, Grandaliano G, Van Kooten C. Kidney Transplantation and Innate Immunity. Lausanne, Switzerland: Frontiers Media SA; 2020

[4] Lambris JD, Holers M, Ricklin D. Complement Therapeutics. New York, USA: Springer Science; 2012

[5] Lefaucheur C. Complement activation in kidney transplantation: From risk stratification to therapeutic strategies. Clinical and Experimental Immunology. 2014;**178**(Suppl. 1):57-58. DOI: 10.1111/cei.12511

[6] Regele H, Bohmig GA. Tissue injury and repair in allografts: Novel perspectives. Current Opinion in Nephrology and Hypertension. 2003;**12**(3):259-266. DOI: 10.1097/00041552-200305000-00006

[7] MacMillan S, Hosgood S, Rahfeld P, Walker-Panse L, Macdonald SS, Kizhakkedathu N, et al. O232: Enzymatic blood group conversion prevents complement activation in an ABO-incompatible model of human kidney transplantation. British Journal of Surgery. 2024;**111**(suppl. 2):1. DOI: 10.1093/bjs/znae046.009

[8] Golshayan D, Schwotzer N, Fakhouri F, Zuber J. Targeting the complement pathway in kidney transplantation. Journal of the American Society of Nephrology. 2023;**34**(11):1776-1792. DOI: 10.1681/ASN.0000000000000192

[9] Valenzuela NM, Hickey MJ, Reed EF. Antibody subclass repertoire and graft outcome following solid organ transplantation. Frontiers in Immunology. 2016;**7**:1-19. DOI: 10.3389/fimmu.2016.00433

[10] Obrecht A, Olagne J, Meuleman MS, Keller N, Chauvet S, Roumenina L, et al. Assessment of in situ alternative and classical convertases as indicators of ongoing glomerular complement activation in IgA nephropathy. Nephrology, Dialysis, Transplantation. 2024;**39**(Suppl. 1):i534-i535. DOI: 10.1093/ndt/gfae069.312

[11] Hresko S, Madarova M, Dobosova M, Palusekova N, Niznerova P, Ziaran S, et al. The diagnostic significance of C4d deposits, as an immunohistochemical proof of complement activation, in kidney glomerular pathologies and kidney transplantation. Bratislavské Lekárske Listy. 2024;**125**(5):275-280. DOI: 10.4149/BLL_2024_41

[12] Stacks S. The Effects of Renal Cold Storage and Transplantation on Immunoproteasome and the Complement System. Arkansas, USA: Scholarly Commons @ Ouachita; 2020

[13] Duval A, Obrecht A, Meuleman MS, Durey MAD, Gautier-Vargas G, Cognard N, et al. Plasma complement activation profile in kidney transplant recipients with IgAN supports the importance of the complement alternative pathway in IgAN. Nephrology, Dialysis, Transplantation. 2024;**39**

(Suppl. 1):i580-i581. DOI: 10.1093/ndt/gfae069.341

[14] Tringali E, Vetrano D, Tondolo F, Maritati F, Fabbrizio B, Pasquinelli G, et al. Looking for a new role of known players: The additional value of plasmatic C3 and C4 in predicting IgA nephropathy prognosis, an observational study. Nephrology, Dialysis, Transplantation. 2024;**39**(Suppl. 1):i567-i569. DOI: 10.1093/ndt/gfae069.335

[15] Prokopenko EI. Atypical hemolytic-uremic syndrome: Evolution of treatment and impact of clinical and genetic characteristics on possibility of eculizumab withdrawal. Nephrology (Saint-Petersburg). 2022;**26**(3):19-29. DOI: 10.36485/1561-6274-2022-26-3-19-29

[16] Yerigeri K, Kadatane S, Mongan K, Boyer O, Burke LL, Sethi SK, et al. Atypical hemolytic-uremic syndrome: Genetic basis, clinical manifestations, and a multidisciplinary approach to management. Journal of Multidisciplinary Healthcare. 2023;**16**:2233-2249. DOI: 10.2147/JMDH.S245620

[17] Dorr CR, Guan W, Onyeaghala G, Oetting WS, Mannon RB, Agarwal G, et al. 487 digital spatial profiling of allograft loss in kidney biopsies with chronic allograft dysfunction. Journal of Clinical and Translational Science. 2024;**8**(Suppl. 1):144. DOI: 10.1017/cts.2024.413

[18] Zheng L, Rong R, Wang X, Li L. Role of the immune system in renal transplantation: Importance, mechanism, and therapy. Frontiers in Immunology. 2024:156

[19] Bernuy-Guevara C, Chehade H, Muller YD, Vionnet J, Cachat F, Guzzo G, et al. The inhibition of complement system in formal and emerging indications: Results from parallel one-stage pairwise and network meta-analyses of clinical trials and real-life data studies. Biomedicine. 2020;**8**(9):355. DOI: 10.3390/biomedicines8090355

[20] Thomas KA, Valenzuela NM, Gjertson D, Mulder A, Fishbein MC, Parry GC, et al. An anti-C1s monoclonal, TNT003, inhibits complement activation induced by antibodies against HLA. American Journal of Transplantation. 2015;**15**(8):2037-2049. DOI: 10.1111/ajt.13273

[21] Noris M, Remuzzi G. Overview of complement activation and regulation. Seminars in Nephrology. 2013;**33**(6):479-492. DOI: 10.1016/j.semnephrol.2013.08.001

[22] Bartoli G, Strologo AD, Grandaliano G, Pesce F. Updates on C3 glomerulopathy in kidney transplantation: Pathogenesis and treatment options. International Journal of Molecular Sciences. 2024;**25**(12):6508. DOI: 10.3390/ijms25126508

[23] Moldakhmetova S, Ali S, Sheerin N. Hypoxia induces complement activation on human kidney epithelial cells. Nephrology, Dialysis, Transplantation. 2023;**38**(Suppl. 1):i202-i203

[24] Kepska M, Chomicka I, Karakulska-Prystypiuk E, Tomaszewska A, Basak G, Zorawski M, et al. Increased urinary biomarkers of kidney injury in patients after allogenetichematopoetic stem cell transplantation reflect kidney damage even in normal kidney function. Nephrology, Dialysis, Transplantation. 2020;**35**(Suppl. 3):i944

[25] Losappio V, Franzin R, Infante B, Godeas G, Gesualdo L, Fersini A, et al. Molecular mechanisms of premature aging in hemodialysis: The complex interplay between innate and adaptive immune dysfunction. International

Journal of Molecular Sciences. 2020;**21**(10):3422. DOI: 10.3390/ijms21103422

[26] Hau HM, Jahn N, Vlachos C, Eichler T, Lederer A, Geisler A, et al. Does timepoint of surgical procedure affect the outcome in simultaneous pancreas-kidney transplantation? A retrospective single-center analysis over 20 years. Journal of Clinical Medicine. 2024;**13**(13):3688. DOI: 10.3390/jcm13133688

[27] Yerly P, Rotman S, Regamey J, Aubert V, Aur S, Kirsch M, et al. Complement blockade with eculizumab to treat acute symptomatic humoral rejection after heart transplantation. Xenotransplantation. 2022;**29**(1):e12726. DOI: 10.1111/xen.12726

[28] Castellano G, Franzin R, Stasi A, Divella C, Sallustio F, Pontrelli P, et al. Complement activation during ischemia/reperfusion injury induces pericyte-to-myofibroblast transdifferentiation regulating peritubular capillary lumen reduction through pERK signaling. Frontiers in Immunology. 2018;**9**:1002. DOI: 10.3389/fimmu.2018.01002

[29] Mehra NK, Baranwal AK, Tait BD. Antibody repertoire and graft outcome following solid organ transplantation. Frontiers in Immunology. 2017:178

[30] Rath T. Current Issues and Future Direction in Kidney Transplantation. London, UK: IntechOpen; 2013

[31] Moise A, Baston C, Cucu N, Ursu LD, Iacob MM, Constantinescu I. Challenges and clinical significance of virtual crossmatch in kidney transplantation: Our experience. SM Journal of Urology. 2017;**3**(3):1032. DOI: 10.36876/smju.1032

[32] Munoz-Herrera CM, Gutierrez-Bautista JF, Lopez-Nevot MA. Complement binding anti-HLA antibodies and the survival of kidney transplantation. Journal of Clinical Medicine. 2023;**12**(6):2335. DOI: 10.3390/jcm12062335

[33] Elshair HS, Naga SS, Ahmed MA, Hanno AY. Influence of donor complement component allotype on renal transplantation outcome. Journal of the Egyptian Society of Nephrology and Transplantation. 2023;**23**(1):26-32

[34] Thongprayoon C, Hansrivijit P, Leeaphorn N, Acharya P, Torres-Ortiz A, Kaewput W, et al. Recent advances and clinical outcomes of kidney transplantation. Journal of Clinical Medicine. 2020;**9**(4):1193. DOI: 10.3390/jcm9041193

[35] Nieuwenhuijs-Moeke GJ, Pischke SE, Berger SP, Sanders JSF, Pol RA, Struys MMRF, et al. Ischemia and reperfusion injury in kidney transplantation: Relevant mechanisms in injury and repair. Journal of Clinical Medicine. 2020;**9**(1):253. DOI: 10.3390/jcm9010253

[36] De Latour RP, Risitano AM. Complement inhibition in medicine: Hematology and beyond; complement inhibition in hematology: PNH and beyond. American Journal of Hematology. 2023;**98**(Suppl. 4):S3-S4. DOI: 10.1002/ajh.26912

[37] Lammerts R. Novel Approaches in Complement Profiling; Application in Kidney Transplantation. Groningen, Netherlands: University of Groningen Press; 2022

[38] Lambris JD, Mastellos DC, Reis ES. Therapeutic modulation of the complement system: Clinical indications and emerging drug leads. Frontiers in Immunology. 2020:185

[39] Liu BC, Lan HY, Lv LL. Renal Fibrosis: Mechanisms and Therapies. Singapore: Springer; 2019

[40] Okumi M. Editorial comment to administration of adipose stromal vascular fraction attenuates acute rejection in donation after circulatory death rat renal transplantation. International Journal of Urology. 2022;**29**(3):275-276. DOI: 10.1111/iju.14773

[41] Chen J, Tsim KWK, Zhao YY. Applications of herbal medicine to control chronic kidney disease: Volume II. Frontiers in Pharmacology. 2022;**13**:1086049. DOI: 10.3389/fphar.2022.1086049

[42] Hara H, Sahara H, Chen-Yoshikawa TF. Future directions for xenotransplantation in lungs. Current Opinion in Organ Transplantation. 2024;**29**(5):332-339. DOI: 10.1097/MOT.0000000000001161

[43] Kesarwani V, Bukhari MH, Kahlenberg JM, Wang S. Urinary complement biomarkers in immune-mediated kidney diseases. Frontiers in Immunology. 2024;**3**(15):1357869. DOI: 10.3389/fimmu.2024.1357869

Chapter 6

What Is the Role of Surgery in Secondary and Tertiary Hyperparathyroidism?

Diana Vetter and Thomas Schachtner

Abstract

Secondary hyperparathyroidism (sHPT) contributes significantly to renal osteodystrophy, cardiovascular morbidity, and mortality. Pharmacological management includes phosphate-lowering treatments for persistent overt hyperphosphatemia, calcitriol and vitamin D analogs for hypocalcemia, and less frequent calcimimetics. Refractory sHPT, unresponsive to pharmacological treatments, necessitates an individualized approach to parathyroidectomy (PTx). PTx in refractory sHPT should be considered when parathyroid hormone levels progressively rise or sHPT-related symptoms persist. Subtotal PTx or total PTx with auto-transplantation is preferred for patients eligible for kidney transplantation. For those not considered for kidney transplantation, total PTx is an option. Additional thymectomy, mainly when the lower parathyroid glands cannot be located, may be performed. Tertiary hyperparathyroidism (tHPT) frequently persists at two years of follow-up after kidney transplantation. THPT often involves multiple glands, adversely affecting bone metabolism, cardiovascular risk, and kidney allograft function, thus warranting PTx. Subtotal PTx remains the preferred surgical approach. When glandular autonomy is suspected, the timing of PTx ideally precedes kidney transplantation. If PTx is required post-kidney transplantation, most centers delay surgery until one year after transplantation to improve kidney allograft outcomes. The decision for PTx and its extent and timing must be carefully individualized, balancing the risks and benefits to maximize patient outcomes in both sHPT and tHPT.

Keywords: parathyroidectomy, tertiary hyperparathyroidism, secondary hyperparathyroidism, CKD-MBD, extent of parathyroidectomy, timing of parathyroidectomy

1. Introduction

The parathyroid glands are the primary regulators of calcium metabolism. Calcium plays a crucial role in nerve conduction, muscle contraction, and bone mineralization, underscoring the importance of the parathyroid glands. In secondary hyperparathyroidism (sHPT), the elevated serum parathyroid hormone (PTH) levels are not due to a malfunction within the parathyroid glands themselves. Instead, low serum calcium levels stimulate all parathyroid glands. Potential causes include vitamin D deficiency and chronic kidney disease (CKD), conditions where 25(OH) vitamin D is not converted to its active form, $1,25(OH)^2$ calcitriol. SHPT is a major contributor to chronic kidney disease-mineral and bone disorder (CKD-MBD) [1]. CKD-MBD is a complex syndrome seen in CKD patients that includes renal osteodystrophy, disturbances in mineral metabolism, and cardiovascular disease [1]. Depending on the stage of CKD, the prevalence of sHPT ranges from 20 to 80% [2–4]. SHPT further increases the risk of vascular and valvular calcification [5, 6] and is associated with high cardiovascular morbidity and mortality in non-dialysis and dialysis patients [7–10].

Refractory sHPT is characterized by progressively rising and persistently elevated PTH levels that do not adequately respond to medical treatments, such as phosphate-lowering treatments, calcitriol and vitamin D analogs, and calcimimetics, without causing hyperphosphatemia or hypercalcemia. In patients who experience improved glomerular filtration rate (GFR) following kidney transplantation, abnormalities in calcium, phosphate, and vitamin D metabolism often normalize, allowing PTH levels to return to physiological levels gradually. However, prolonged stimulation of the parathyroid glands can lead to tertiary hyperparathyroidism (tHPT), characterized by a persistent elevation of PTH due to parathyroid autonomy, resulting in mild to moderate hypercalcemia and hypophosphatemia. THPT after kidney transplantation has been found to impact bone quality negatively [11, 12], reduce kidney allograft function and survival [13], and increase cardiovascular and overall mortality [13].

This book chapter will focus on the pathophysiology of sHPT and tHPT and its treatments, particularly emphasizing the current surgical practices, including the extent and timing of parathyroidectomy (PTx).

2. Definition and pathogenesis of secondary and tertiary hyperparathyroidism

In advanced CKD, hyperphosphatemia, hypocalcemia, and decreased $1,25(OH)^2$ calcitriol levels cause continuous stimulation of the parathyroid glands via direct and indirect mechanisms. This results in increased PTH production and release [14]. Persistently elevated PTH levels increase serum calcium levels through three primary mechanisms: First, PTH enhances vitamin D activation to $1,25(OH)^2$ calcitriol, thereby improving intestinal calcium absorption. Second, PTH reduces renal calcium excretion, and third, PTH increases serum calcium levels by promoting bone resorption.

In the last decade, this understanding has been augmented by the discovery of the fibroblast growth factor 23 (FGF23), a phosphaturic protein produced in osteocytes and osteoblasts with multiple effects. FGF23 is stimulated early in CKD, preceding clinically evident hyperphosphatemia [15]. Together with the cofactor/coreceptor Klotho, which facilitates FGF23 binding to the FGF23 receptors in the kidneys, parathyroid glands, and bone, phosphate excretion is increased through different mechanisms: First, FGF23 increases renal phosphate excretion in the proximal tubule, second it decreases PTH excretion in the parathyroid glands, and third it inhibits vitamin D activation in the kidney [15]. However, in advanced CKD, the phosphaturic capacity of FGF23 becomes exhausted, so elevated FGF23 levels indirectly stimulate PTH and contribute to the progression of sHPT [15].

Ultimately, sHPT is characterized by (1) normal or decreased serum calcium levels, depending on the compensatory capacity of the parathyroid glands; (2)

increased serum phosphate and FGF23 levels, and (3) decreased 1,25(OH)^2 calcitriol levels. Refractory sHPT is defined by progressively rising and persistently elevated PTH levels that do not adequately respond to medical treatments, such as phosphate-lowering treatments, calcitriol and vitamin D analogs, and calcimimetics, without resulting in significant hyperphosphatemia or hypercalcemia.

If end-stage CKD, as the cause of sHPT, is corrected by kidney transplantation, abnormalities in calcium, phosphate, and vitamin D metabolism often normalize, and PTH levels gradually return to physiological levels. However, it is assumed that in many individuals, the normalization of kidney function following kidney transplantation does not lead to the normalization of parathyroid function. SHPT has been shown to decrease from 70% at one year to 43% at two years after kidney transplantation [16]. Long-term stimulation of the parathyroid glands in CKD can lead to gland hyperplasia, and over time, polyclonal stimulation may result in nodular remodeling. From this point, somatic mutations can lead to predominantly monoclonal proliferation with reduced sensitivity of the calcium-sensing and vitamin D receptors on the parathyroid cells. At this stage, parathyroid cells no longer undergo normal regulation and do not respond to typical PTH-suppressive stimuli such as normalized serum calcium levels. Consequently, serum calcium levels rise, and parathyroid autonomy develops, a condition known as tHPT. Although the clinical manifestations of hypercalcemia and hypophosphatemia resemble primary hyperparathyroidism, multiglandular disease is common in tHPT.

3. Impact of secondary hyperparathyroidism on chronic kidney disease: Mineral and bone disorder

Clinically, patients with sHPT exhibit various signs and symptoms, primarily impacting the bone with bone and joint pain and incident fractures and the cardiovascular system with extra-skeletal calcifications of vasculature and valves and, in rare cases soft tissue resulting in calciphylaxis [17].

The decreased levels of 1,25(OH)^2 calcitriol in CKD lead to deficient bone mineralization, known as *osteomalacia*. Conversely, the PTH-stimulating effect enhances bone turnover, decreasing laminar bone and increasing trabecular bone volume, a condition termed *osteitis fibrosa cystica*. When bone turnover is reduced due to medical treatment, this is called *adynamic bone disease*. All three forms of skeletal involvement—*osteomalacia*, *osteitis fibrosa cystica*, and *adynamic bone disease*—are common in CKD and collectively known as renal osteodystrophy [11, 18]. Unlike osteoporosis, where trabecular bone is primarily affected, renal osteodystrophy predominantly impacts cortical bone [18]. PTH increases bone volume but not the mass of trabecular bone, leaving the mechanically strong lamellar bone less affected. An iliac crest biopsy remains the gold standard for diagnosing and classifying renal osteodystrophy. While bone mineral density (BMD) assessments by dual-energy X-ray absorptiometry (DXA) are designed to evaluate osteoporosis and are not ideal for assessing renal osteodystrophy, they are less invasive. Therefore, low and declining BMD, in combination with increasing serum alkaline phosphatase levels, used as indicators of elevated bone turnover, are reasonable biomarkers to predict incident fracture risk in CKD patients with renal osteodystrophy and to support the use of osteoporosis medications [19].

In addition to renal osteodystrophy, sHPT is associated with high cardiovascular morbidity and mortality [8–10, 13]. Given that most patients with sHPT have elevated phosphate levels, it cannot be excluded that hyperphosphatemia contributes significantly to the high cardiovascular risk. In addition, elevated FGF23 levels in advanced CKD have deleterious effects on vascular and valvular calcification [20], and left ventricular hypertrophy (LVH), putting those patients at the highest cardiovascular risk.

This complex syndrome associated with CKD is termed CKD-MBD [17, 21]. It encompasses mineral metabolism abnormalities, bone abnormalities (renal osteodystrophy), and vascular calcification. SHPT is the predominant driver of CKD-MBD.

4. Medical treatment options for secondary hyperparathyroidism and tertiary hyperparathyroidism

The only causative treatment for refractory sHPT in patients with CKD is kidney transplantation. All other treatments aim to improve dysregulation and reduce morbidity, serving as symptomatic treatments. General recommendations for CKD patients on dialysis are to maintain PTH levels in the range of approximately two to nine times the upper normal limit of the assay (i.e., 585 pg./mL if the upper range of normal is 65 pg./mL). PTH levels of around 300 pg./mL are considered compensatory and represent an appropriate adaptive response due to phosphaturic effects and increasing bone resistance to PTH. Patients with progressively rising and persistently elevated PTH levels, alongside hyperphosphatemia or hypercalcemia despite optimized medical treatment, are considered refractory, and PTx may be evaluated [21]. In addition to optimizing dialysis dose and adequacy, medical treatments include phosphate-lowering treatments, calcitriol and vitamin D analogs, calcimimetics, or a combination thereof.

4.1 Phosphate-lowering treatments

High phosphate levels are associated with increased mortality in advanced CKD patients (CKD 3a-5) [9]. This has led to the widespread use of phosphate-restrictive diets and phosphate binders in CKD patients. However, phosphate-lowering treatments may suppress PTH, potentially leading to adynamic bone disease. Calcium-based phosphate binders may increase vascular and valvular calcification [22], and aluminum-containing phosphate binders have shown toxicity due to aluminum accumulation [23]. Despite the clear association between high phosphate levels and mortality, there is no proof that phosphate restriction or phosphate-lowering treatments improve cardiovascular morbidity. Consequently, the use of phosphate-lowering treatments has become more restrictive, particularly calcium-based preparations, with the recommendation to treat hyperphosphatemia only if phosphate levels are repeatedly high (e.g., above 1.8 mmol/L) and not to treat CKD patients prophylactically [21].

4.2 Calcitriol and vitamin D analogs

In advanced CKD patients, low levels of $1{,}25(OH)^2$ calcitriol stimulate parathyroid glands due to decreased intestinal calcium uptake and subsequent serum calcium drop, suggesting vitamin D supplementation as a potential solution. Two randomized controlled trials (RCTs) examined the effects of calcitriol or vitamin D analogs on cardiac endpoints [24, 25], revealing a significant increase in hypercalcemia without beneficial effects on surrogate cardiac endpoints. Given the morbidity associated with hypercalcemia and the related increase in phosphate and FGF23 levels, the risk-benefit ratio of treating moderate PTH elevations using calcitriol or vitamin D analogs is not clearly favorable. Routine use of calcitriol or vitamin D analogs is not recommended and should be reserved for severe and progressive sHPT, administered in low doses titrated based on PTH response while avoiding hypercalcemia [19].

4.3 Calcimimetics

Calcimimetics such as cinacalcet allosterically activate the calcium-binding site of PTH receptors in the parathyroid glands, lowering PTH and calcium levels, often resulting in hypocalcemia. In a well-designed RCT with 3383 dialysis patients randomized to either calcimimetics or placebo, calcimimetics significantly reduced PTH levels without affecting mortality, non-fatal cardiovascular events, or fracture rate [26, 27]. This has led to discussions about whether cinacalcet should be a first-line option for all patients with sHPT and advanced CKD requiring PTH-lowering treatment. Currently, there is no clear recommendation, but calcimimetics remain an option when PTH is markedly elevated and resulting mild hypocalcemia could be tolerated [21]. The potential of newer calcimimetic agents to reduce PTx rates among dialysis patients remains uncertain. In dialysis patients, the intravenous calcimimetic etelcalcetide has been shown to lower PTH levels more effectively than cinacalcet [9, 14].

4.4 Bone-directed therapies

Renal osteodystrophy encompasses three main forms: osteomalacia, osteitis fibrosa cystica, and adynamic bone disease with low bone turnover. Adynamic bone disease, which is particularly detrimental, should be avoided if possible. Low bone turnover can be disease-related (e.g., malnutrition, diabetes, and hyperphosphatemia in CKD leading to PTH hyporesponsiveness) or triggered by medical treatments [28]. Specifically, calcium supplementation, calcitriol, vitamin D analogs, calcimimetics, and PTx can lead to adynamic bone disease due to over-suppression of PTH in the parathyroid glands [28]. Bone-directed treatments aim to shift the bone mineral balance toward a positive state, including antiresorptive and osteoanabolic treatments. Antiresorptive therapies inhibit osteoclasts, which cause bone resorption as counterplayers to osteoblasts. As antiresorptive agents, bisphosphonates induce osteoclast apoptosis, while denosumab decreases osteoclast development. Both are associated with atypical femur fractures and are not recommended for adynamic bone disease or hypocalcemic patients, as they can exacerbate hypocalcemia. They may be considered in patients with high bone turnover, weighing the risk of antiresorptive use against the accuracy of diagnosing the underlying bone phenotype.

Abaloparatide and romosozumab, as osteoanabolic agents, offer the benefit of stimulating osteoblast activity, which can be particularly advantageous in addressing adynamic bone disease with low bone turnover. However, their use must be carefully monitored to prevent potential complications such as hypercalcemia. Achieving a balance between their anabolic effects and minimizing the risk of exacerbating adynamic bone disease is crucial for optimizing patient outcomes.

5. The indication for parathyroidectomy in secondary hyperparathyroidism and its potential benefits

If medical treatment cannot control severe refractory sHPT, PTx must be evaluated. According to the KDIGO guidelines, this is indicated when PTH remains progressively rising and persistently above nine times the normal range despite treatment with calcitriol, vitamin D analogs, calcimimetics, or a combination thereof [21]. However, PTx is rarely performed at this level in the absence of sHPT-related symptoms such as bone and joint pain, myopathy, or severe extra-skeletal calcifications.

The German guidelines recommend starting with a phosphate-lowering treatment if phosphate levels are repeatedly elevated (e.g., above 1.8 mmol/l). If PTH rises above 300 pg./mL, vitamin D analogs or calcimimetics should be administered. Vitamin D analogs are preferred in hypocalcemic patients to correct vitamin D deficiency. At the same time, calcimimetics can be an option in hypercalcemic patients, although the KDIGO 2017 does not explicitly recommend their use. If these medical treatments and optimizing dialysis dose and adequacy are unsuccessful, PTx may be recommended [1].

However, the indication for PTx must be individualized based on factors such as age, cardiovascular risk, other comorbidities, and preparation for possible kidney transplantation. In severely symptomatic patients, the indication for PTx exists independent of these factors. In asymptomatic patients, while there is no consensus on a PTH level that mandates PTx, progressively rising PTH levels above 1000 pg./mL may be considered an indication.

The rationale is clear: elevated PTH levels significantly raise morbidity by increasing cardiovascular risk, incident fracture risk, and overall mortality. Therefore, removing the source of PTH production should mitigate these effects.

Regarding renal osteodystrophy, a matched retrospective study on nearly 6000 hemodialysis patients showed that PTx reduced the risk of hip fractures by 32% [29]. This could be because patients with PTx experienced less pain and, therefore, moved more freely, positively impacting bone strength. Another study examined cardiovascular mortality in over 114,000 hemodialysis patients in Japan. In over 4000 hemodialysis patients matched with just as many who underwent PTx, not having had a PTx was a risk factor for all-cause and cardiovascular mortality [7].

In terms of future kidney allograft function, Callender et al. retrospectively examined 900 kidney transplant recipients, 57 of whom had a PTx before transplantation. They found that a six-fold increase in PTH at the time of transplantation was associated with kidney allograft loss. PTx before transplantation was associated with a lower risk of kidney allograft loss [30].

Additionally, PTx has been shown to significantly improve symptoms in patients with primary, sHPT, and tHPT. Patients with sHPT had the most prominent symptoms and were not entirely symptom-free after surgery. Symptom improvement in patients with primary and tHPT was similar. Symptoms were measured using the median symptom index score (MSIS), which includes 13 items, such as bone pain, depressive mood, and memory impairments [31]. For sHPT, symptom improvement after PTx was confirmed in another study using the parathyroidectomy assessment of symptoms (PAS) score [32].

PTx in patients with sHPT has notable perioperative morbidity. Besides the small risk of recurrent laryngeal nerve palsy and bleeding, mortality is increased in the postoperative period. A study of over 4500 hemodialysis patients with PTx, compared with just as many without PTx, showed that mortality was significantly higher in the PTx group until 90 days postoperatively. However, after 587 days, the mortality risk decreased for patients who underwent PTx [33]. Thus, while perioperative mortality is higher, long-term mortality is lower in hemodialysis patients who undergo PTx.

Overall, PTx in patients with refractory sHPT appears to benefit bone integrity, cardiovascular morbidity, and mortality, particularly in dialysis patients, and may also impact future kidney allograft survival.

6. Parathyroidectomy for secondary hyperparathyroidism

Various surgical options are available when discussing PTx for sHPT. These include (1) total PTx with resection of all four parathyroid glands with auto-transplantation, (2) total PTx without auto-transplantation, and (3) subtotal PTx, which involves leaving half of the most normal-looking gland *in situ*. Additionally, a thymectomy can be performed as part of the procedure. Determining the optimal treatment requires careful consideration of multiple studies comparing these surgical approaches. Some studies compare total PTx with auto-transplantation to subtotal PTx [34–36], while others compare total PTx with or without auto-transplantation (**Table 1**), [39–42].

In summary, (1) subtotal PTx has the lowest hypoparathyroidism rate but the highest reoperation rate due to recurrence or persistence. (2) Total PTx with auto-transplantation has a higher hypoparathyroidism rate than subtotal PTx but a lower

Publication	Study design	Compared groups	Outcome
Schneider et al. [37]	Retrospective	• Total PTx + AT (n = 504) • Subtotal PTx (n = 32) • Total PTx -AT (n = 21) • Incomplete PTx (n = 49)	PTx-AT: • Lowest recurrence, ns • Lowest persistence, ns
Isaksson [38]	Retrospective Sweedish registry data	• Total PTx (n = 388) • Subtotal PTx (n = 436)	Subtotal PTx: • Lower kardiovascular risk • Higher risk for recurrence
Chen et al. [34]	Systematic review and meta-analysis (13 studies, n = 1589)	• Total PTx + AT (n = 1064) • Subtotal PTx (n = 621)	• Recurrence ns • Persistence ns • Reoperation rate ns
Rothmund et al. [35]	**RCT**	• Subtotal PTx (n = 20) • Total PTx + AT (n = 20)	PTx + AT: • Clinical improvement ↗
Yuan et al. [36]	Systematic review and meta-analysis (18 studies, n = 3656)	• Subtotal PTx (n = 1864) • Total PTx + AT (n = 1792)	ns: • Symptoms • Hypocalcemia rate • Persistence • Recurrence • Reoperation rate Total PTx + AT • Prolonged in-hospital stay • Serum calcium 1 mo FU ↘
Schlosser et al. [39]	**Multicenter prosp. RCT**	• Total PTx + AT + thymectomy (n = 48) • Total PTx (n = 52)	Total PTx + AT+thymectomy at 3 y FU • Calcium ns, PTH levels ↗ • Recurrence ↗ (8.3% vs. 0% without AT)

Publication	Study design	Compared groups	Outcome
Jia et al. [40]	Meta-analysis (7 cohort studies, n = 931)	• Total PTx + AT (n = 621) • Total PTx –AT (n = 150) • Other PTx (n = 160)	Total PTx-AT • Persistence↘ • Recurrence ↘ • Reoperation rate↘
Li et al. [41]	Meta-analysis (10 cohort studies, 1 RCT; n = 1108)	• Total PTx + AT (n = 833) • Total PTx-AT (n = 275)	• Hypoparathyroidism rate↗ • No patients recorded with severe hypocalcemia or adynamic bone disease
Liu et al. [42]	Meta-analysis (9 cohort studies, 1 RCT; n = 1283)	• Total PTx + AT • Total PTx-AT	

Table 1.
Studies on extent of parathyroidectomy in sHPT.

need for potentially less challenging reoperations. (3) Total PTx without autotransplantation has the lowest reoperation rate but the highest risk of postoperative hypoparathyroidism (**Table 2**). This lower reoperation rate advantage comes at the cost of a greater lifelong need for calcium supplementation, risk of tetany, and risk of adynamic bone disease due to low PTH levels.

Interestingly, patients undergoing subtotal PTx seem to have a lower cardiovascular risk and may have better kidney allograft function than those undergoing total PTx. Hypocalcemia and a significant PTH drop are detrimental to kidney allograft function. Studies indicate hypocalcemia and pronounced PTH drops are risk factors for decreased kidney allograft function [43]. Patients with no parathyroid tissue left will have lower serum calcium levels and a more significant PTH drop. Since PTH has a vasodilatory effect on preglomerular vessels and a potent action on renal plasma flow [44], a pronounced PTH drop after PTx may lead to reduced renal plasma flow and acute deterioration of kidney function. However, long-term animal studies suggest that treating sHPT might protect the kidney from the progression of chronic renal failure despite the acute risks associated with PTH drops post-PTx [45, 46].

	Subtotal PTx	Total PTx + AT	Total PTx - AT
Postoperative hypocalcemia	↘	→	→
Reoperation rate	↗	→	→
Persistence and Recurrence	→	→	↘
Advantages	• Cardiovascular risk↘[1] • Graft function[2] ↗	• Morbidity of revisional surgery risk↘	• Persistence ↘ • Recurrence ↘
Disadvantages	• Cervical seeding • Morbidity of revisional surgery↗	• Longer postoperative hypocalcemia • Seeding at implantation localization	• Lifelong calcium substitution • Risk for tetany↗ • Risk for adynamic bone disease↗

[1]*Isaksson et al. [38].*
[2]*Schwarz et al. [43].*

Table 2.
Advantages and disadvantages of different parathyroidectomy extents in sHPT.

The current recommendation for CKD patients with severe refractory sHPT and an indication for PTx is to leave some parathyroid tissue behind, especially in patients who are or might be listed for kidney transplantation, to potentially enable normal parathyroid function and avoid hypoparathyroidism. In elderly patients without the option of kidney transplantation, total PTx without auto-transplantation can be considered. Since the lower parathyroid glands can lie within the thymus in up to 39% of patients [37, 47], a thymectomy is indicated whenever the lower parathyroid gland cannot be found and can also be performed routinely to reduce persistency or recurrence rates. It might even be recommended for patients who will never be transplanted.

7. The indication for parathyroidectomy in tertiary hyperparathyroidism and its potential benefits

SHPT can resolve with PTH normalization in approximately 30% of cases within one year and 57% within two years after kidney transplantation [16]. However, almost 50% of patients develop parathyroid autonomy, known as tHPT, which often leads to mild or moderate hypercalcemia. This condition is considered irreversible, even when the glomerular filtration rate (GFR) remains normalized in the long-term post-kidney transplantation. Unlike patients with sHPT undergoing dialysis, kidney transplant recipients generally do not exhibit severe symptoms, as tHPT is less severe.

What impact does tHPT have after kidney transplantation (**Table 3**)? Similar to primary hyperparathyroidism, elevated PTH levels in kidney transplant recipients

tHPT associated morbidity	Study	Study design	Results
Renal Osteodystrophy	Heaf et al. [11]	Retrospective, 3 years FU, n = 114 • Assoc. between MBD und PTH	PTH > 150 ng/L decreases bone density significantly
	Perrin et al. [12]	Retrospective, n = 143 KTRs • Risk factors for fractures after kidney Tx	Elevated PTH after Kidney Tx is significant risk factor for fracture rate • 8% after 1 year • 15% after 2 years
Graft function	Gwinner et al. [48]	Retrospective, n = 213 KTRs • Kidney biopsies at 6 weeks, 3 and 6 months after Tx	tHPT after Kidney Tx correlates with • Graft calcifications within 6 months • Decreased graft function
Mortality	Lou et al. [16]	Retrospective, n = 1609 KTRs • PTH normalization at 1 and 2 years after Tx • Graft- and overall survival	Early PTH normalization after Kidney Tx improves Graft- and overall survival
	Pihlstrom et al. [13]	Retrospective, n = 2102 KTRs; mean FU 5.1 years Association between PTH and • Cardiovascular events • Graft loss and mortality	PTH > 65 pg./ml: • 85% higher risk of graft loss ($p < 0.001$) • 46% higher risk of mortality ($p = 0.006$)

KTRs = Kidney transplant recipients.

Table 3.
Morbidity associated with tHPT in kidney transplant recipients.

negatively affect bone density. A PTH level above 150 pg./mL, three times the normal level, has been shown to decrease bone density significantly [11]. Additionally, elevated PTH levels increase the fracture rate. The fracture incidence was 8% one year and as high as 15% two years post-transplantation if PTH levels remained elevated [12]. Persisting tHPT has also been shown to increase kidney allograft calcification within six months post-transplantation, associated with worse kidney allograft function [48]. Other studies have confirmed decreased kidney allograft function in the presence of tHPT [13, 16]. In one study, 43% of patients with persistent HPT two years after kidney transplantation had lower kidney allograft survival and overall patient survival, prompting the authors to advocate for early surgical intervention post-transplantation [16]. Pihlstrom et al. found an 85% increased risk of kidney allograft loss and a 46% higher mortality risk when PTH levels were above 65 ng/L (**Table 3**), [13]. However, the exact mechanism by which tHPT contributes to kidney allograft loss still remains unknown.

Can elevated PTH levels after kidney transplantation be positively affected by PTx (**Table 4**)? Few studies have investigated the morbidity of kidney transplant recipients based on whether they had a PTx. Collaud et al. found improved bone mineral density in kidney transplant recipients after PTx compared to before PTx in a small patient sample [49]. Additionally, PTx for tHPT may benefit kidney allograft function in the mid to long term. However, a significant drop in PTH and subsequent hypocalcemia can be detrimental to kidney allograft function [43]. Other studies have reported deterioration of kidney allograft function after PTx [39, 51]. In a retrospective study comparing 100 kidney transplant recipients with tHPT treated with the calcimimetic cinacalcet to 33 patients treated with PTx, those treated with PTx had a higher rate of PTH normalization and significantly lower kidney allograft loss (**Table 4**), [50]. Despite representing an additional perioperative risk to kidney allograft function, treating tHPT with PTx benefits kidney allograft function in the long-term post-transplantation.

Given the limited data on the indications for PTx in kidney transplant recipients with tHPT, decisions must be individualized based on factors such as age, cardiovascular risk, other comorbidities, the success of the kidney transplantation, and long-term prognosis. Although symptoms of tHPT are usually mild to moderate, the improvement of symptoms [31] and the long-term benefit for kidney allograft function may justify PTx in in a greater number of patients.

tHPT associated morbidity	Study	Study design	Improvement by PTx?
Renal Osteodystrophy	Collaud et al. [49]	Retrospective, PTx after Kidney Tx for tHPT n = 14, mean FU 26 months • BMD before- and after PTx	PTx significantly increased BMD ($p < 0.01$)
Graft function	Finnerty et al. [50]	Retrospective Graft function in KTRs with tHPT n = 133, median FU 7 years • Cinacalcet (n = 100) • subtotal PTx and bilateral thymectomy (n = 33)	PTx • PTH normalization ↗ • Graft-failure ↘ (9% vs. 33%, p = 0.007)

Table 4.
Effect of PTx for tHPT in kidney transplant recipients.

8. Parathyroidectomy for tertiary hyperparathyroidism

To determine the optimal extent of PTx for tHPT, it is essential to understand that 90% of tHPT patients present with multiglandular disease, with only 10% affected by a single parathyroid gland and 30% by two glands.

Ideally, only the autonomous parathyroid glands would be removed to maintain self-regulated calcium homeostasis. Achieving this requires excellent localization methods or a thorough four-gland exploration to identify and remove abnormal parathyroid glands. To date, no such ideal localization diagnostic exists. Sonography can localize enlarged parathyroid glands with a low sensitivity of around 62% for sHPT and tHPT [52]. Despite its limitations sonography remains important in renal hyperparathyroidism, also to exclude coexisting thyroid pathologies before parathyroid surgery. The sensitivity of scintigraphy for renal hyperparathyroidism is low (around 55%) [52]. To date, the Choline-PET /MRI or Choline-PET/CT is the best imaging modality with the highest specificity (93%) and sensitivity (86%) for detecting hyperplastic parathyroid glands in patients with secondary and tertiary HPT [52]. Data for Choline-PET in renal HPT is however still scarce, so that a recommendation for its regular use in renal HPT cannot yet be given. The four-gland exploration remains the best localization method for autonomous parathyroid glands in renal HPT. However, normal appearing glands may still be autonomous, and many patients may experience advanced CKD anew, again leading to stimulation of the parathyroid glands and potentially necessitating additional surgery.

There are no prospective randomized controlled trials (RCTs) on the ideal surgical approach for tHPT. In a multicenter retrospective study, 61 kidney transplant recipients who underwent subtotal PTx were compared to 44 kidney transplant recipients who underwent total PTx with auto-transplantation. At six months follow-up, the hypoparathyroidism rate was significantly lower in the subtotal PTx group, while the cure rate was the same in both groups [53]. The authors concluded that subtotal PTx was superior to total PTx with auto-transplantation in kidney transplant recipients.

The question remains whether less than subtotal PTx might be sufficient for kidney transplant recipients with tHPT. Data in this area is sparse and inconsistent. One retrospective study with 19 kidney transplant recipients who underwent less than subtotal PTx and 52 kidney transplant recipients who underwent subtotal PTx found no differences in recurrence rates. The transient hypocalcemia rate was higher in the subtotal group, but no patient experienced permanent hypocalcemia. The authors concluded that the more focused procedure had the same success rate as subtotal PTx [54]. This conclusion, however, is debated. Triponez et al. retrospectively examined a similar patient set with 83 kidney transplant recipients who received subtotal or less than subtotal PTx, removing only the enlarged glands. After a mean follow-up of 5.4 years, the group with less than subtotal surgery had a 5.2 times higher risk of persistent or recurrent disease, leading Triponez et al. to recommend against less than subtotal surgery [55].

Currently, most endocrine surgeons will explore all four glands and perform a subtotal PTx for tHPT.

9. Timing for parathyroidectomy

The timing of PTx in relation to kidney transplantation has been investigated retrospectively. A study analyzing 190 kidney transplant recipients examined three time points: PTx before kidney transplantation, PTx within one year after kidney transplantation, and PTx more than one year after kidney transplantation [56]. The findings indicated that undergoing PTx after kidney transplantation was associated with decreased kidney allograft function. Specifically, if PTx was performed after kidney transplantation, the GFR dropped post-surgery. For kidney transplant recipients who underwent PTx within one year of kidney transplantation, kidney allograft function did not recover, whereas if PTx was performed more than one year after kidney transplantation, kidney allograft function improved. Based on these results, the authors concluded that PTx should ideally be performed before kidney transplantation if parathyroid autonomy is suspected. If hyperparathyroidism persists after kidney transplantation, PTx should not be performed within one year to protect the graft [56].

Contradicting these findings, another study demonstrated that early post-transplantation PTx (within 278 days) for patients with tHPT was associated with significantly better kidney allograft function compared to late referral (after 278 days) in a small cohort (n = 19 vs. 19) [57]. This data, along with evidence of kidney graft calcification within 6 months of kidney transplantation if hyperparathyroidism persists, supports earlier surgical intervention for tHPT.

10. Conclusion

The differentiation between sHPT and tHPT is critical, especially when it comes to surgical interventions by PTx. For refractory sHPT, PTx becomes necessary when medical therapies fail, offering significant benefits in reducing cardiovascular morbidity and mortality and improving bone integrity. On the other hand, tHPT often develops post-kidney transplantation, where prolonged stimulation of the parathyroid glands leads to parathyroid autonomy. Surgical intervention for tHPT, particularly subtotal PTx, is crucial to enhance kidney allograft function and mitigate complications such as hypercalcemia, cardiovascular risk, and bone density loss. The surgical indication for PTx, extent, and timing must be carefully individualized according to the patient's age, cardiovascular risk, other comorbidities, and the overall prognosis. Balancing the risks and benefits to optimize patient outcomes in both sHPT and tHPT remains challenging but should be evaluated more liberally concerning PTx.

Conflict of interest

The authors declare no conflict of interest.

Acronyms and abbreviations

sHPT	secondary hyperparathyroidism
PTH	parathyroid hormone
FGF23	fibroblast growth factor 23
CKD	chronic kidney disease
tHPT	tertiary hyperparathyroidism
CKD-MBD	chronic kidney disease-mineral bone disorder
BMD	bone mineral density
LVH	left ventricular hypertrophy
PTx	parathyroidectomy
GFR	glomerular filtration rate

Author details

Diana Vetter[1*] and Thomas Schachtner[2]

1 Department of Abdominal Surgery and Transplantation, University Hospital of Zurich, Zurich, Switzerland

2 Department of Nephrology, University Hospital of Zurich, Zurich, Switzerland

*Address all correspondence to: diana.vetter@usz.ch

References

[1] Kidney Disease: Improving Global Outcomes CKDMBDWG. KDIGO clinical practice guideline for the diagnosis, evaluation, prevention, and treatment of chronic kidney disease-mineral and bone disorder (CKD-MBD). Kidney International. 2009;**113**:S1-S130

[2] Bureo JC, Arevalo JC, Anton J, Adrados G, Jimenez Morales JL, Robles NR, et al. Prevalence of secondary hyperparathyroidism in patients with stage 3 and 4 chronic kidney disease seen in internal medicine. Endocrinología y Nutrición. 2015;**62**(7): 300-305

[3] Levin A, Bakris GL, Molitch M, Smulders M, Tian J, Williams LA, et al. Prevalence of abnormal serum vitamin D, PTH, calcium, and phosphorus in patients with chronic kidney disease: Results of the study to evaluate early kidney disease. Kidney International. 2007;**71**(1):31-38

[4] Andress DL, Coyne DW, Kalantar-Zadeh K, Molitch ME, Zangeneh F, Sprague SM. Management of secondary hyperparathyroidism in stages 3 and 4 chronic kidney disease. Endocrine Practice. 2008;**14**(1):18-27

[5] Horl WH. The clinical consequences of secondary hyperparathyroidism: Focus on clinical outcomes. Nephrology, Dialysis, Transplantation. 2004;**19** (Suppl. 5):V2-V8

[6] Kamycheva E, Sundsfjord J, Jorde R. Serum parathyroid hormone level is associated with body mass index. The 5th Tromso study. European Journal of Endocrinology. 2004;**151**(2):167-172

[7] Komaba H, Taniguchi M, Wada A, Iseki K, Tsubakihara Y, Fukagawa M. Parathyroidectomy and survival among Japanese hemodialysis patients with secondary hyperparathyroidism. Kidney International. 2015;**88**(2):350-359

[8] De Boer IH, Gorodetskaya I, Young B, Hsu CY, Chertow GM. The severity of secondary hyperparathyroidism in chronic renal insufficiency is GFR-dependent, race-dependent, and associated with cardiovascular disease. Journal of the American Society of Nephrology. 2002;**13**(11):2762-2769

[9] Block GA, Klassen PS, Lazarus JM, Ofsthun N, Lowrie EG, Chertow GM. Mineral metabolism, mortality, and morbidity in maintenance hemodialysis. Journal of the American Society of Nephrology. 2004;**15**(8):2208-2218

[10] Ganesh SK, Stack AG, Levin NW, Hulbert-Shearon T, Port FK. Association of elevated serum PO(4), Ca x PO(4) product, and parathyroid hormone with cardiac mortality risk in chronic hemodialysis patients. Journal of the American Society of Nephrology. 2001; **12**(10):2131-2138

[11] Heaf J, Tvedegaard E, Kanstrup IL, Fogh-Andersen N. Hyperparathyroidism and long-term bone loss after renal transplantation. Clinical Transplantation. 2003;**17**(3):268-274

[12] Perrin P, Caillard S, Javier RM, Braun L, Heibel F, Borni-Duval C, et al. Persistent hyperparathyroidism is a major risk factor for fractures in the five years after kidney transplantation. American Journal of Transplantation. 2013;**13**(10):2653-2663

[13] Pihlstrom H, Dahle DO, Mjoen G, Pilz S, Marz W, Abedini S, et al. Increased risk of all-cause mortality and renal graft loss in stable renal transplant

recipients with hyperparathyroidism. Transplantation. 2015;**99**(2):351-359

[14] Cunningham J, Locatelli F, Rodriguez M. Secondary hyperparathyroidism: Pathogenesis, disease progression, and therapeutic options. Clinical Journal of the American Society of Nephrology. 2011;**6**(4):913-921

[15] Donate-Correa J, Muros-de-Fuentes M, Mora-Fernandez C, Navarro-Gonzalez JF. FGF23/klotho axis: Phosphorus, mineral metabolism and beyond. Cytokine & Growth Factor Reviews. 2012;**23**(1–2):37-46

[16] Lou I, Foley D, Odorico SK, Leverson G, Schneider DF, Sippel R, et al. How well does renal transplantation cure hyperparathyroidism? Annals of Surgery. 2015;**262**(4):653-659

[17] Uhlig K, Berns JS, Kestenbaum B, Kumar R, Leonard MB, Martin KJ, et al. KDOQI US commentary on the 2009 KDIGO clinical practice guideline for the diagnosis, evaluation, and treatment of CKD-mineral and bone disorder (CKD-MBD). American Journal of Kidney Diseases. 2010;**55**(5):773-799

[18] Parfitt AM, Drezner MK, Glorieux FH, Kanis JA, Malluche H, Meunier PJ, et al. Bone histomorphometry: Standardization of nomenclature, symbols, and units. Report of the ASBMR histomorphometry nomenclature committee. Journal of Bone and Mineral Research. 1987;**2**(6): 595-610

[19] Lorenz K. S2k guideline "surgical therapy of primary and renal hyperparathyroidism". Chirurgie (Heidelb). 2023;**94**(2):176

[20] Budoff MJ, Rader DJ, Reilly MP, Mohler ER 3rd, Lash J, Yang W, et al. Relationship of estimated GFR and coronary artery calcification in the CRIC (chronic renal insufficiency cohort) study. American Journal of Kidney Diseases. 2011;**58**(4):519-526

[21] Ketteler M, Elder GJ, Evenepoel P, Ix JH, Jamal SA, Lafage-Proust MH, et al. Revisiting KDIGO clinical practice guideline on chronic kidney disease-mineral and bone disorder: A commentary from a kidney disease: Improving global outcomes controversies conference. Kidney International. 2015;**87**(3):502-528

[22] Jamal SA, Vandermeer B, Raggi P, Mendelssohn DC, Chatterley T, Dorgan M, et al. Effect of calcium-based versus non-calcium-based phosphate binders on mortality in patients with chronic kidney disease: An updated systematic review and meta-analysis. Lancet. 2013;**382**(9900):1268-1277

[23] Pepper R, Campbell N, Yaqoob MM, Roberts NB, Fan SL. Do oral aluminium phosphate binders cause accumulation of aluminium to toxic levels? BMC Nephrology. 2011;**12**:55

[24] Thadhani R, Appelbaum E, Pritchett Y, Chang Y, Wenger J, Tamez H, et al. Vitamin D therapy and cardiac structure and function in patients with chronic kidney disease: The PRIMO randomized controlled trial. JAMA. 2012;**307**(7):674-684

[25] Wang SM, Kulkarni L, Dolev J, Kain ZN. Music and preoperative anxiety: A randomized, controlled study. Anesthesia and Analgesia. 2002;**94**(6): 1489-1494, table of contents

[26] Investigators ET, Chertow GM, Block GA, Correa-Rotter R, Drueke TB, Floege J, et al. Effect of cinacalcet on cardiovascular disease in patients undergoing dialysis. The New England

Journal of Medicine. 2012;**367**(26): 2482-2494

[27] Moe SM, Abdalla S, Chertow GM, Parfrey PS, Block GA, Correa-Rotter R, et al. Effects of cinacalcet on fracture events in patients receiving hemodialysis: The EVOLVE trial. Journal of the American Society of Nephrology. 2015;**26**(6):1466-1475

[28] Haarhaus M, Evenepoel P, European Renal Osteodystrophy w, Chronic Kidney Disease M, Bone Disorder working group of the European Renal Association-European D, Transplant A. Differentiating the causes of adynamic bone in advanced chronic kidney disease informs osteoporosis treatment. Kidney International. 2021;**100**(3):546-558

[29] Rudser KD, de Boer IH, Dooley A, Young B, Kestenbaum B. Fracture risk after parathyroidectomy among chronic hemodialysis patients. Journal of the American Society of Nephrology. 2007; **18**(8):2401-2407

[30] Callender GG, Malinowski J, Javid M, Zhang Y, Huang H, Quinn CE, et al. Parathyroidectomy prior to kidney transplant decreases graft failure. Surgery. 2017;**161**(1):44-50

[31] Pasieka JL, Parsons LL. A prospective surgical outcome study assessing the impact of parathyroidectomy on symptoms in patients with secondary and tertiary hyperparathyroidism. Surgery. 2000; **128**(4):531-539

[32] Cheng SP, Lee JJ, Liu TP, Yang TL, Chen HH, Wu CJ, et al. Parathyroidectomy improves symptomatology and quality of life in patients with secondary hyperparathyroidism. Surgery. 2014; **155**(2):320-328

[33] Kestenbaum B, Andress DL, Schwartz SM, Gillen DL, Seliger SL, Jadav PR, et al. Survival following parathyroidectomy among United States dialysis patients. Kidney International. 2004;**66**(5):2010-2016

[34] Chen J, Jia X, Kong X, Wang Z, Cui M, Xu D. Total parathyroidectomy with autotransplantation versus subtotal parathyroidectomy for renal hyperparathyroidism: A systematic review and meta-analysis. Nephrology (Carlton, Vic.). 2017;**22**(5):388-396

[35] Rothmund M, Wagner PK, Schark C. Subtotal parathyroidectomy versus total parathyroidectomy and autotrans-plantation in secondary hyperpara-thyroidism: A randomized trial. World Journal of Surgery. 1991;**15**(6):745-750

[36] Yuan Q, Liao Y, Zhou R, Liu J, Tang J, Wu G. Subtotal parathyroidectomy versus total parathyroidectomy with autotransplantation for secondary hyperparathyroidism: An updated systematic review and meta-analysis. Langenbeck's Archives of Surgery. 2019; **404**(6):669-679

[37] Schneider R, Waldmann J, Ramaswamy A, Fernandez ED, Bartsch DK, Schlosser K. Frequency of ectopic and supernumerary intrathymic parathyroid glands in patients with renal hyperparathyroidism: Analysis of 461 patients undergoing initial parathyroidectomy with bilateral cervical thymectomy. World Journal of Surgery. 2011;**35**(6):1260-1265

[38] Isaksson E, Ivarsson K, Akaberi S, Mut A, Prütz KG, Clyne N, et al. Total versus subtotal parathyroidectomy for secondary hyperparathyroidism. Surgery. Jan 2019;**165**(1):142-150. DOI: 10.1016/j.surg.2018.04.076. Epub 2018 Nov 7. PMID: 30413319

[39] Schlosser K, Bartsch DK, Diener MK, Seiler CM, Bruckner T, Nies C, et al. Total parathyroidectomy with routine thymectomy and autotransplantation versus total parathyroidectomy alone for secondary hyperparathyroidism: Results of a nonconfirmatory multicenter prospective randomized controlled pilot trial. Annals of Surgery. 2016;**264**(5): 745-753

[40] Jia X, Wang R, Zhang C, Cui M, Xu D. Long-term outcomes of Total Parathyroidectomy with or without autoimplantation for hyperparathyroidism in chronic kidney disease: A meta-analysis. Therapeutic Apheresis and Dialysis. 2015;**19**(5): 477-485

[41] Li C, Lv L, Wang H, Wang X, Yu B, Xu Y, et al. Total parathyroidectomy versus total parathyroidectomy with autotransplantation for secondary hyperparathyroidism: Systematic review and meta-analysis. Renal Failure. 2017; **39**(1):678-687

[42] Liu ME, Qiu NC, Zha SL, Du ZP, Wang YF, Wang Q, et al. To assess the effects of parathyroidectomy (TPTX versus TPTX+AT) for secondary hyperparathyroidism in chronic renal failure: A systematic review and meta-analysis. International Journal of Surgery. 2017;**44**:353-362

[43] Schwarz A, Rustien G, Merkel S, Radermacher J, Haller H. Decreased renal transplant function after para-thyroidectomy. Nephrology, Dialysis, Transplantation. 2007;**22**(2):584-591

[44] Wolzt M, Schmetterer L, Dorner G, Zelger G, Entlicher J, Kapiotis S, et al. Hemodynamic effects of parathyroid hormone-related peptide-(1-34) in humans. The Journal of Clinical Endocrinology and Metabolism. 1997; **82**(8):2548-2551

[45] Shigematsu T, Caverzasio J, Bonjour JP. Parathyroid removal prevents the progression of chronic renal failure induced by high protein diet. Kidney International. 1993;**44**(1):173-181

[46] Ogata H, Ritz E, Odoni G, Amann K, Orth SR. Beneficial effects of calcimimetics on progression of renal failure and cardiovascular risk factors. Journal of the American Society of Nephrology. 2003;**14**(4):959-967

[47] Uno N, Tominaga Y, Matsuoka S, Tsuzuki T, Shimabukuro S, Sato T, et al. Incidence of parathyroid glands located in thymus in patients with renal hyperparathyroidism. World Journal of Surgery. 2008;**32**(11):2516-2519

[48] Gwinner W, Suppa S, Mengel M, Hoy L, Kreipe HH, Haller H, et al. Early calcification of renal allografts detected by protocol biopsies: Causes and clinical implications. American Journal of Transplantation. 2005;**5**(8):1934-1941

[49] Collaud S, Staub-Zahner T, Trombetti A, Clerici T, Marangon N, Binet I, et al. Increase in bone mineral density after successful parathyroidectomy for tertiary hyperparathyroidism after renal transplantation. World Journal of Surgery. 2008;**32**(8):1795-1801

[50] Finnerty BM, Chan TW, Jones G, Khader T, Moore M, Gray KD, et al. Parathyroidectomy versus cinacalcet in the management of tertiary hyperparathyroidism: Surgery improves renal transplant allograft survival. Surgery. 2019;**165**(1):129-134

[51] Kandil E, Florman S, Alabbas H, Abdullah O, McGee J, Noureldine S, et al. Exploring the effect of parathyroidectomy for tertiary hyperparathyroidism after kidney transplantation. The American Journal of the Medical Sciences. 2010; **339**(5):420-424

[52] Chen YH, Chen HT, Lee MC, Liu SH, Wang LY, Lue KH, et al. Preoperative F-18 fluorocholine PET/CT for the detection of hyperfunctioning parathyroid glands in patients with secondary or tertiary hyperparathyroidism: Comparison with Tc-99m sestamibi scan and neck ultrasound. Annals of Nuclear Medicine. 2020;**34**(8):527-537

[53] Choi SR, Lim JH, Kim MY, Hong YA, Chung BH, Chung S, et al. Cinacalcet improves endothelial dysfunction and cardiac hypertrophy in patients on hemodialysis with secondary hyperparathyroidism. Nephron Clinical Practice. 2012;**122**(1–2):1-8

[54] Nichol PF, Starling JR, Mack E, Klovning JJ, Becker BN, Chen H. Long-term follow-up of patients with tertiary hyperparathyroidism treated by resection of a single or double adenoma. Annals of Surgery. 2002;**235**(5):673-678; discussion 8-80

[55] Triponez F, Kebebew E, Dosseh D, Duh QY, Hazzan M, Noel C, et al. Less-than-subtotal parathyroidectomy increases the risk of persistent/recurrent hyperparathyroidism after para-thyroidectomy in tertiary hyperparathyroidism after renal transplantation. Surgery. 2006;**140**(6): 990-997; discussion 7-9

[56] Littbarski SA, Kaltenborn A, Gwiasda J, Beneke J, Arelin V, Schwager Y, et al. Timing of parathyroidectomy in kidney transplant candidates with secondary hyperparathryroidism: Effect of pretransplant versus early or late post-transplant parathyroidectomy. Surgery. 2018;**163**(2):373-380

[57] Dream S, Chen H, Lindeman B. Tertiary hyperparathyroidism: Why the delay? Annals of Surgery. 2021;**273**(3): e120-e1e2

Section 2

Advances and Future Directions in Kidney Transplantation

Chapter 7

When There Is No Need for Immunosupresives: Combined Bone Marrow and Kidney Transplantation

Vedad Herenda, Damir Rebić, Aida Hamzić-Mehmedbašić, Azra Ribić-Mrkonja and Merima Odobašić

Abstract

The holy grail of transplantation is the induction of donor-specific tolerance. In that possible scenario, there is no need for immunosuppressive therapy anymore. The main goal of this approach is to improve allograft survival by avoiding side effects of immunosuppressive therapy. There are promising reports about patients whose allograft kidney function remains stable after they have undergone bone marrow transplantation. The main obstacle in the last years was too aggressive therapy and procedures that were undertaken before bone marrow transplantation. There is high potential of this approach as well as dangers but due to progress in science, it is reasonable to believe that combined transplantation could be used more in the future.

Keywords: bone marrow and kidney transplantation, allogenic transplantation, tolerance, immunosuppression, chimerism

1. Introduction

At present, kidney transplantation remains the best treatment for patients with terminal-stage chronic kidney disease. Three cornerstones of successful kidney transplantations are vascular anastomosis, short-term hypothermic organ preservation, and inhibition of immune rejection. The first two problems were successfully solved, but the third, immune rejection, remains the biggest and the most complicated challenge. Advancements were made by the introduction of potent immunosuppressive drugs, but new problems arose: susceptibility to infections, the rise of malignant diseases, de novo diabetes, dyslipidemia, neurotoxicity and chronic allograft nephropathy due to the effect of immunosuppressive drugs. Even 1 year of renal allograft survival has dramatically improved during the last decades at 90%; long-term allograft survival has not changed for decades. Third, patients will lose their renal graft in 10 years after transplantation [1]. More depressing is the fact that 50% of renal graft losses are with functioning renal grafts, due to premature death of patients. The most common causes of death in kidney transplant patients are cardiovascular events and cancer [2].

Transplantation tolerance, "the lack of destructive immune responses to a transplanted organ in the absence of immunosuppression," could be a possible answer to these problems [3]. It was first described by Oven in 1945 when he realized that dizygotic bovine twins are tolerant to each other's blood due to placental interchange during gestation. Medawar experimentally induced tolerance in 1953 after experiments with mice just before the first successful kidney transplant on the Herrick twins 1 year later in 1954 by Joseph Murray. Operational tolerance is a term that describes one group of patients in which immunosuppressive therapy was withdrawn intentionally or due to non-adherence, but graft function remained stable for more than 1 year without signs of destruction by the immune system [4].

Avoidance of immunosuppressive therapy is possible only by the induction of transplantation tolerance. So far, the most promising ways to achieve successful transplantation tolerance in humans are regulatory cell therapy and hemopoietic chimerism. Combined bone marrow and kidney transplantation seems to be a promising approach with huge potential for future use. They are first described in patients with multiple myeloma [5].

Estimated lifetime money savings are substantial in those kidney transplant patients with induced tolerance [4]. In wider clinical use, combined kidney and hematopoietic stem cell transplantation (HSCT) transplantation with developed tolerance will improve renal allograft's long-term survival as well as the quality of life of patients opening a new chapter in transplant medicine.

2. Concept of tolerance and resistance in transplantation medicine

Medical professionals from the very beginning were trying to resolve autoimmune response complications, or so-called graft versus host disease (GvHD). Transplant recipients are still in need of life-long chronic immunosuppression, which results in drug-specific side effects and complications due to suppression of the host immune response. Under long-term immunosuppression, the patient is at risk of neoplastic, infectious, and cardiovascular complications, which can implicate a shortened life and a functional renal graft. Some other morbidities include nephrotoxicity, neurotoxicity, de novo diabetes mellitus iatrogenic, and dyslipidemia. All these complications could be controlled, reduced, or completely avoided if successful immunologic tolerance was induced, and that is why, this is supposed to be the main goal in transplantation medicine.

Upon exposure to a foreign antigen, either the antigen is eliminated by the standard immune response of the host – or so-called resistance – or the immune system adapts to the pathogen, promoting immune tolerance instead.

Self-tolerance, the ability not to destroy itself, may be induced in immature self-reactive lymphocytes in generative lymphoid organs – called central tolerance – or in mature lymphocytes in peripheral sites – called peripheral tolerance.

There are two obligatory elements for achieving transplantation tolerance: depletion of alloreactive T conventional cells and upregulation of T regulatory cells. In patients with solid organ transplantations, at the transplantation time – it is discovered that there are more alloantigen-reactive T conventional cells in the recipient compared with the relatively small number of T regulatory cells, which means that the balance of cells is shifted toward allograft destruction. Achieving balance between graft destruction and regulation/tolerance can be done using strategies to inhibit the activity of T conventional cells and/or increase the relative frequency or functional activity of alloantigen-reactive T regulatory cells. According to previous, mixed chimeric and cellular tolerogenic therapies are being the element of research in transplantation tolerance.

Very important to mention are the significant complication in transplantation medicine – graft versus host disease, the state where the immune cells from transplanted tissue recognize the recipient's body as foreign and attack its cells. The immune system's cells are being learned early to differentiate between self and foreign cells. The ability to recognize nonself/foreign cells depends on the histocompatibility genes, which provide instructions for making a group of related proteins known as major histocompatibility complex proteins or HLA. During transplantation, the donor tissue prompts immune cells in the graft to recognize the recipient's HLA proteins as nonself, triggering an immune response between the donor and the recipient. Mismatched organs, or organs that are not matched closely enough, can trigger a transplant rejection.

Tolerance in transplantation medicine is supposed to be the most important thing in coexisting in solid organ transplantation. This phenomenon of immune tolerance, where there is no response to foreign tissues, according to the literature, was first described by Ray D. Owen in 1945, when he discovered mixed chimerism in the freemartin cattle. He noted that dizygotic twin cattle sharing a common placenta also shared a stable mixture of each other's red blood cells. His study showed the body could be tolerant of foreign tissues. In 1953, Leslie Brent, Rupert E. Billingham, and Peter Medawar showed that by injecting foreign cells into fetal or neonatal mice, they could eventually accept future grafts from the same foreign donor. Sir Frank McFarlane Burnet and Frank Fenner were the first to propose the deletion of self-reactive lymphocytes to establish tolerance, now termed clonal deletion, and it was the next step in improving the idea of immunotolerance.

In 1978, at Stanford University, the research group reported successful induction of skin allograft tolerance in mice using persistent chimerism established by total lymphoid irradiation. Based on these animal studies, they proceeded with a clinical trial using total lymphoid irradiation and rabbit anti-thymocyte globulin, but without donor bone marrow transplantation, and reported successful induction of renal allograft tolerance.

Kawai and his colleagues have developed a non-myeloablative conditioning regimen to induce renal allograft tolerance in non-human primates. Splenectomy and a brief course of cyclosporine are supposed to be necessary for the induction of mixed chimerism. Renal allograft tolerance was reproducibly achieved with the induction of only transient mixed chimerism. In this research, the conditioning regimen was subsequently improved by replacing splenectomy with either anti-CD154 mAb or belatacept. Translating these models to a clinical protocol to induce renal allograft tolerance in HLA-mismatched kidney transplantations has shown impressive results. The regimen included cyclophosphamide (60 mg/kg), thymic irradiation (7 Gy), humanized anti-CD2 mAb with or without rituximab, and posttransplant calcineurin inhibitors. Patients developed transient mixed chimerism for 1–3 weeks without graft vs. host disease, and 70% of patients have successfully achieved immunosupressive-free survival 5 years afterwards. As an adverse event associated with this approach, transient acute kidney injury was observed after combined kidney bone marrow transplantation in nine of the 10 recipients.

In clinical practice, according to the data in the literature, the first evidence of tolerance through hematopoietic stem cell transplantation was described by Sayegh in 1991, who had a case of a 30-year-old man diagnosed with acute myelomonocytic leukemia and a 14-year-old girl with acute nonlymphocytic leukemia. Both received hematopoietic stem cell transplantation from their HLA-identical brothers. After a few years and gradual loss of their renal function, their donors agreed to also donate a kidney. Except for small maintenance doses of steroids, no immunosuppression was given in the further course, and the kidney function of the transplant remained stable. According to this research, more cases were described in the literature afterward.

In our nephrological world, achieving transplantation tolerance completely without losing functional graft would be the most important goal for our patients, the community, and medical professionals.

2.1 Mechanisms of self and transplantation tolerance, cellular and molecular base, and dysfunction

The human immune system has great potential for the creation of sensory receptors and thus gains the ability to neutralize all antigens that enter the body as foreign bodies. The high possibility of sensitization by antibodies leads to the activity of the immune response and its high specificity for antigens. There are two types of immune response: non-specific – innate immune response – and specific – acquired immune response. In addition to defense against infection, the primary role is the maintenance of gene and antigen homeostasis. This is preceded by the ability of the immune system to distinguish its own from foreign antigens. Against its antigens, it initiates a tolerance reaction, and against foreign antigens, an immune reaction that fights and expels the foreign pathogen/antigen from the body. Acquired immunity includes the recognition of antigens and the activation of a specific reaction, as well as the development of the immunological memory of T lymphocytes and B lymphocytes. First, the primary receptors on B and T lymphocytes are activated, which activate the central lymphatic tissue, namely, B lymphocytes in the bone marrow and T lymphocytes in the thymus, as a late immune response activation of peripheral lymphatic tissue (spleen and lymph nodes) occurs. T lymphocytes recognize the antigen in the form of a peptide bound to the MHC protein (MHC-major histocompatibility complex), and B lymphocytes use immunoglobulin receptors with which they can recognize parts of the antigen called antigenic epitopes.

Innate and acquired immune responses are closely related. Antigen-specific activation of T lymphocytes activates the production of cytokines and chemokines that activate components of innate immunity, as well as specific mechanisms of antibody production and cytotoxicity mediated by CD8+ cells. These reactions also include the production of complement components, which are necessary for a complete immune response.

Given that the transplanted organ (kidney, bone marrow, etc.) is never completely genetically identical to the donor, there is a great chance of developing an immune (transplantation) response. The aforementioned reaction is directed primarily toward ABO blood group antigens, foreign HLA molecules, and tissue antigens such as the H antigen. These belong to antigens of the minor histocompatibility complex (MHC-minor histocompatibility complex). The intensity of the transplant response depends on several factors: the degree of HLA matching, antigen-presenting cells, and the presence of antibodies in the recipient's serum that could have been created by earlier sensitization (receiving blood products). HLA antigens are among the strongest transplantation antigens that represent the target of immune and transplantation activity. They are encoded by two groups of MHC genes – MHC I and MHC II, which are characterized by polygeny and polymorphism. Polygeny shows the fact that similar genes encode protein products that perform the same function. Polymorphism refers to the fact that one of the larger number of different alleles found in the general human population can appear at each of the mentioned gene loci. During the evaluation, HLA molecules became extremely polymorphic and can bind a large number of peptides to microorganisms, thereby providing immunity against most infections. This fact is precisely the cause of strong transplant alloreactivity because future HLA molecules not only play a role in antigen presentation but also become transplant antigens that trigger an immune response in the recipient. On HLA antigens, we find different epitopes (certain sequences of amino acids) with which antibodies can react. We find common epitopes on different HLA antigens. Due to this fact, the matching of HLA antigen epitopes to which donor-specific antibodies (DSA – donor-specific antibodies) bind is very important in transplantation.

Based on this, it is concluded that, in transplantation, the fact of epitope matching of HLA antigens is more important than the overall matching in the constellation of the HLA system, which can reduce the formation of DSA and increase the number of acceptable organs and improve the post-transplantation outcome.

Sometimes, a transplant reaction can develop even in the case of ideal HLA matching between the donor and recipient of the organ. It takes place on the grounds of differences in the secondary syngenes of concordance, and the reaction of rejection takes place through the indirect path of rejection. Hyperacute rejection as a result of anti-HLA antibodies is extremely strong today; however, donor-specific antibodies that occur cause poor graft survival due to acute or chronic antibody-induced rejection reactions. This humoral rejection is often followed by T-lymphocyte-mediated rejection (cell-type rejection). where B lymphocytes are activated after recognizing the B-lymphocyte receptor with the help of the CD4+ subtype of T lymphocytes. The binding of the B-cell receptor to the antigen leads to the formation of an antigen-receptor complex, which creates endosomes, and then phagoendosomes, where the antigen is broken down into peptides. The resulting peptides bind to the HLA class II molecule and return to the B-lymphocyte membrane by endosomal transport. The HLA molecules shown in this way are recognized by CD4+ helper T lymphocytes, and B lymphocytes receive the first signal of activation. CD4 + T lymphocytes also secrete cytokines necessary for the differentiation of B lymphocytes into plasma cells or memory B lymphocytes.

Plasma cells migrate to the bone marrow, and memory cells to secondary lymphatic tissues, which ensures long-term specific humoral immunity. Plasma cells, as the final products of B lymphocyte differentiation, after their contact with an antigen, produce antibodies – immunoglobulins (IgM, IgA, IgE, and IgG). Antibodies have a part called an Fc fragment on them, which they can use to bind to those cells that have an Fc receptor. The most common association with the antigen is mediated by IgG antibodies, so that as the target cells in the transplanted organ, the antibodies damage the transplanted organ in two ways, through the activation of the classical complement pathway and binding of effector cells through the Fc fragment.

Complement activation itself acts chemotactically and anaphylactically, and ultimately cytotoxic, and this mechanism contributes to chronic rejection of the transplanted organ. Antibodies have an affinity toward the endothelium, through the mediation of the Fc fragment on the antibodies, and the greatest damage to the transplanted organ is caused by macrophages, although other cells with this fragment can also participate in the cellular cytotoxicity reaction mediated by antibodies. Thanks to certain markers on B lymphocytes, they can be demonstrated in the biopsy of a transplanted organ, and by direct action on them, they reduce or stop the immune response.

2.2 Regulatory immune cells in transplantation-new insights and developments of drug

The population of leukocytes can have double roles: promoting rejection or tolerance. Innate immune cells are macrophages/monocytes, natural killer cells, neutrophils, mast cells, eosinophils, dendritic cells, and myeloid-derived suppressive cells. Differentiation of macrophages into pro-inflammatory M1 and anti-inflammatory M2 types has a role in promoting acute and chronic rejection of transplanted organs or prolonging graft survival through suppressive mechanisms. Natural killer cells are a vital part of the innate immune system and play a role in the surveillance of tumors, viruses, and fungi. In transplantation, they can promote T-cell-mediated rejection by up-regulating pro-inflammatory cytokines, promoting DC maturation, and marking donor tissue for destruction. They could induce tolerance by inhibiting alloreactive T cells and antigen-presenting cells (APCs), directly killing donor-derived DCs, and inhibiting immune responses. Dendritic cells are crucial for antigen presentation and connect innate and adaptive immune systems with the activation of B and T cells. Neutrophils react to damage-associated molecular patterns (DAMPs), triggering oxidative stress and enzyme release, exacerbating ischemia-reperfusion injury (IRI). They take part in acute and chronic graft rejection through mechanisms such as superoxide production, enzyme release, and formation of neutrophil extracellular traps (NETs). Mast cells participate in graft rejection through several mechanisms: degranulation, cytokine secretion, and activation of fibroblasts. On the other side, mast cells could inhibit T-cell proliferation through interactions with regulatory T cells (Tregs) process mediated by cytokine secretion. Eosinophiles have a role in hypersensitivity reactions and antiparasitic responses. In allograft rejection, they release cytokines such as IL-2. Elevated eosinophil count in peripheral blood and graft tissue correlates with acute rejection. Myeloid-derived suppressive cells (MDSCs) have immunosuppressive properties. They could inhibit immune responses by direct suppression of effector cells and secretion of immunosuppressive cytokines and enzymes [6]. The "T-cell centric" paradigm in the field for decades promoted the main role of T lymphocytes in graft rejection. But, even after T-cell blockade, there is still allograft rejection ongoing which says that there is something more that promotes the reaction of rejection by the innate immune system.

The main adaptive immune cells are B and T lymphocytes. They are essential to protect from malignant and infectious diseases. Also, they could play a role in autoimmune diseases and inflammatory states. Lymphocytes react with precision, and B cells were traditionally considered antibody-producing cells. Donor-specific antibody (DSA) production is one of the B cells' functions the most known in transplant medicine described in 60s by Patel and Terasaki [7]. Antibody-mediated rejection, a process drive by B cells, is the main factor of chronic graft failure. But beside antibody-producing function, B cells have an impact on immune system response through antigen presentation, cytokine production, and co-stimulation.

Effects of B-cells on the immune system is the summation of opposing activity of different subsets of B cells: those with regulatory activity Breg cells or those with effector activity Beff cells [8] Patients who developed operational tolerance have shown a higher frequency of Breg. This B-cell subset affects innate as adaptive system as well through the production of different mechanisms: production of IL-10, IL-35, TGF-β, and IL-35. Through the activity of IL-10, Bregs prevents the proliferation of CD4 + T cells and suppresses CD8+ effector T-cell function. Through binding the FAS and PD-1 receptor, they induce T-cell apoptosis [9]. A specific marker or group of markers to define Bregs as a unique cell subset has not been found so far and that is the new goal of researchers.

T cells were for decades studied due to their central role in transplant graft rejection. That event is classified as either antibody-mediated rejection (AMR) or acute cellular rejection (ACR). ACR is a T-cell-mediated response to the presence of nonself major histocompatibility antigen (MHC). $CD8^+$ cytotoxic T cells are a key effector subset that plays a central role in the destruction of renal allograft after activation. T cells recognize MHC antigens by two signals. The first is provided by antigen presented by MHC which interacts with T-cell receptor (TCR) and second in T-cell and antigen-presenting cells surface (APC). $CD4^+$ cells play a central role in ACR. After activation, they differentiate in different subsets, which are Th17, Th9, Th22, T follicular helper (Tfh), T follicular regulatory (Tfr), and regulatory T-cell (Treg) lineages [10]. The last ones are crucial for maintaining immune tolerance by down-regulating allograft rejection. Also, they have a vital role in preventing autoimmune disease and limiting anti-tumor response. Tregs inhibit immune response and promote tissue recovery. Two main subsets of Treg are thymic-origin (tTreg) and peripherally induced (pTreg) Treg cells. Both subsets are characterized by the presence of CD25 (a chain of IL-2 receptor), low levels of CD127 (IL-7 receptor), and factor Forkhead Box 3 FOXP3 [11, 12]. They constitute a very discreet proportion of $CD4^+$ cells, 5–10% of all subset. FOXP3 gene is located on the X-chromosome. The FOXP3 protein is a 431 amino acid structure with four domains: an amino-terminal proline-rich domain, a central zinc finger, leucine zipper domains, and the C-terminal forkhead domain [12]. It is the master transcription factor of Tregs and strongly regulates their function.

Cell therapies were presented as a new approach to induce tolerance after solid organ transplantation. Mesenchymal stromal/stem cell therapy was at the forefront due to its immunomodulatory and regenerative actions [13]. Due to knowledge of Breg induction and/or expansion, stability, and functional potential, the cell therapy approach using Breg is not yet possible. On the other side, Treg cell therapy studies have shown promising results. In 2016, Todo et al. [14] showed operational tolerance in recipients of living-related liver donors by infusion enriched by donor-specific Tregs. This study was the first of its kind to demonstrate the successful discontinuation of an immunosuppressive regimen due to the effect of Treg-based therapy. Chandran et al. presented their experience with patients with subclinical kidney graft inflammation in a 6-month follow-up period after transplantation who got an infusion of Treg with promising results. The TRACT trial used Treg in de novo kidney transplant patients in 2018 [15]. From 2012 to 2018, the ONE study included eight centers in Europe and the United States. The main goal was to develop a unified approach to cell therapy for patients with solid organ transplants. In his study, six different regulatory cell subsets (four Treg cell products) were evaluated. In the first year, patients had fewer infectious complications, but the rejection rate was similar [16].

Promising results from studies with cell therapy show that regulatory cell therapy is an achievable option and safe option in patients with transplanted kidneys. The use of this therapy will ease the burden of general immunosuppressive and its complications.

3. Induction of chimerism by myeloablative conditioning and bone marrow and kidney transplant, principles of tolerance

To achieve tolerance, durable chimerism is necessary [17]. The term "chimerism" describes a state in which donor hematopoietic cells are present in the recipient organism. It could be achieved by allogeneic bone marrow transplantation (BMT) or allogeneic hematopoietic stem cell transplantation (HSCT) [3]. In terms of forms of chimerism, it could be full or mixed. Full is the replacement of host cells by donor lymphohematopoietic elements. Due to the high risk of graft versus host disease (GvHD), it was not regarded as a possible approach in patients without underlying malignancy.

Mixed chimerism means the presence of both donor and recipient cells [18]. Also, in terms of duration of chimerism, there are persistent-long lasting chimerism over time and transient chimerism with short-term detectability of donor-derived hematopoietic cells [19].

Three centers in the US and one in Korea use different approaches for chimerism induction, as shown in **Table 1**.

To achieve any type of chimerism, a precondition regime is necessary.

Myeloablative regimens are way of treatment in which high-dose total irradiation is used in combination with chemotherapeutic drugs. At the same time, this approach carries the biggest risks of developing complications: infections and graft versus host disease (GvHD). The determining factor for the development of GvHD is a type of chimerism. Persistent full chimeras have more risk of developing GvHD than persistent mixed chimeras. Also, later, they have more advantages over full chimers: the precondition regime is less toxic, and full chimeras have impaired immune responses. However, establishing persistent mixed chimerism is a huge challenge in clinical surroundings and is hard to achieve in HLA-mismatched [5].

In the absence of malignant disease, the risk of GvHD is not justified, as already mentioned. The non-myeloablative regimen was developed by Kawai et al. for renal allograft tolerance in non-human primates, which consists of low-dose total body irradiation (TBI), TI, and anti-T-cell antibody [20]. Also, in those non-myeloablative protocols, thymic irradiation or total lymph node irradiation could be used with different medications afterward. The goal of all of these approaches is to prevent the recurrence of GvHD while preserving renal allograft tolerance at the same time.

The presence of kidney allograft is necessary for the induction and maintenance of tolerance, a state of unresponsiveness of the immune system to specific tissues or cells. There are central and peripheral tolerance mechanisms that are not fully understood so far. The tolerization process depends on the posttransplant evolution of donor and host immune cells. Intrathymic deletion of reactive T cells and the development of new non-reactive cells are the bases of the central tolerance mechanism.

Type of chimerism	HLA match	Center
Persistent mixed chimerism	HLA matched	Stanford
Transient mixed chimerism	HLA mismatched	MGH, SMC
Persistent full chimerism	HLA mismatched	Northwestern University

MGH, Massachusetts General Hospital; SMC, Samsung Medical Center.

Table 1.
Chimerism strategy.

On the opposite side, peripheral tolerance is the summation of three activities: clonal deletion of T-donor-specific cells, peripheral exhaustion, and gradual expansion of induced regulatory T cells (Tregs).

Sustained tolerance is quite a variable process that does not depend on just one factor. It is the result of different cellular and non-cellular activities, some of which are not fully understood so far. Its full understanding in the future will lead to better results in the maintenance and development of new drugs, with the ultimate goal of getting rid of immunosuppressive medications.

4. Solid organ transplantation outcome after bone marrow transplantation: challenges and obstacles

Combined transplantation is a unique challenge. Immunosuppression could lead to the development of end-stage organ failure and malignancies, which require a second transplant. The outcome of patients with combined transplantation will depend on several factors: (i) histocompatibility of the first and second transplanted organ and (ii) sensitivity of solid organ graft to conditioning regime necessary for HCT and effects of long-term immunosuppression, infection complications, and relapse rate after HCT [1]. Acute myeloid leukemia develops in 0.2% of recipients of solid organs. In 1–3% of patients with liver and kidney and 3–9% of heart and lung with up to 10% of intestinal or multiorgan transplants develop posttransplant lymphoproliferative disease (PTLD) [21] Donor of hematopoietic stem cell (HSC) is usually HLA matched with the recipient, not the transplanted organ. Therefore, therefore, alloSCT can lead to graft rejection. If the donor of stem cells and kidney solid organs have the same tolerance, it could develop.

Studies with combined transplantation are scarce, and results are sporadically reported [22]. The European Society for Blood and Marrow Transplantation centers reported on 28 patients with combined transplantation: 12 patients with kidney, 13 with liver, and 3 with heart transplants. Among these patients' solid organ graft failure was 25% at 3 months and 32.8% at 12 months. Patients with a transplanted kidney were more prone to organ failure compared to those with liver transplants. The overall survival (OS) was 75% at 3 months, 60.2% at 12 months, 45.1% at 36 months, and 40.1% at 60 months mostly due to mortality in the first year. Mortality was not caused by relapse of malignancy but due to infection-related complications. The second most common cause of death was the loss of transplant function. Loss of transplant function was more often observed in patients with kidney transplants than in liver grafts and did not influence survival [23].

A study from Japan reported on 19 patients with combined hematopoietic stem cell transplantation (HSCT) and solid organ transplantation: 10 with liver transplantation and 9 with kidney transplant. Eight of all kidney transplant patients experienced renal dysfunction during and after HSCT, with worsening of renal function within 1 year after transplantation. All of them required dialysis, and three of them experienced rejection of renal allograft. Five of nine patients died within the first year after HSCT. In this study, 5-year OS in patients undergoing allo-HSCT was 41.7% for non-malignant disease but just 23.1% for those with malignant disease. Median survival time was 10.7 months for all patients [24]. French study presented excellent overall survival of 94% over 5-year period with excellent kidney graft survival [25].

Although combined kidney-HSCT seems to have promising results, it also has some serious obstacles. Limited availability of donors and different criteria for HSCT and kidney transplants are just some of them [26]. Wider clinical use will depend on the development of less toxic conditioning regimes and prevention of infectious complications as well as cell therapy introduction.

5. Conclusions

Transplantation medicine has had a few breakthrough events in the past: the first successful kidney transplantation and the introduction of cyclosporine are just some of them. The development of donor-specific tolerance will be the next big event in medical history. Promising results were shown by combined kidney and stem cell transplantation. It is limited to a few centers and highly selected patients but shines light on the quest for transplantation without the burden of immunosuppressive drugs. Scarce studies and different data about preconditioning regimens, graft survival, and outcomes necessitate international cooperation for the common good. Potential benefits should overcome all boundaries and differences.

Donor-specific tolerance by the combined kidney and HSC transplantation or by using cell therapy will mark a new age in transplantation. The negative effect of immunosuppressive medications will be minimized, and kidney graft survival will be prolonged for years. All of these will give a new quality of life to kidney transplant patients but, at the same time, open new chapters of the newly described complications and adverse effects of therapy.

Conflict of interest

The authors declare no conflict of interest.

Author details

Vedad Herenda[1,2]*, Damir Rebić[1,3], Aida Hamzić-Mehmedbašić[1,3], Azra Ribić-Mrkonja[1] and Merima Odobašić[1]

1 Clinic for Nephrology Clinical Center University of Sarajevo, Sarajevo, Bosnia and Herzegovina

2 Medical Faculty Sarajevo School of Science and Technology, Sarajevo, Bosnia and Herzegovina

3 Medical Faculty University of Sarajevo, Sarajevo, Bosnia and Herzegovina,

*Address all correspondence to: vedad.herenda@gmail.com

References

[1] Hariharan S, Israni AK, Danovitch G. Long-term survival after kidney transplantation. The New England Journal of Medicine. 2021;**385**:729-743

[2] Wekerle T, Segev D, Lechler R, Oberbauer R. Strategies for long-term preservation of kidney graft function. Lancet. 2017;**389**(10084):2152-2162. DOI: 10.1016/S0140-6736(17)31283-7

[3] Podestà MA, Sykes M. Chimerism-based tolerance to kidney allografts in humans: Novel insights and future perspectives. Frontiers in Immunology. 2021;**12**:791725

[4] Salisbury EM, Game DS, Lechler RI. Transplantation tolerance. Pediatric Nephrology. 2014;**29**(12):2263-2272. DOI: 10.1007/s00467-013-2659-5. Epub 2013 Nov 10

[5] Nayak L, Lazarus H. Renal allografts in plasma cell myeloma hematopoietic cell graft recipients: On the verge of an explosion?. Bone Marrow Transplant. 2013;**48**:338-345. DOI: 10.1038/bmt.2012.111

[6] Xiaojie G, Jian G, Zheng J, Ling L. Diverse roles of immune cells in transplant rejection and immune tolerance. Engineering. 2022;**10**:44-56. ISSN 2095-8099. DOI: 10.1016/j.eng.2021.03.029

[7] Patel R, Terasaki PI. Significance of the positive crossmatch test in kidney transplantation. The New England Journal of Medicine. 1969;**280**:735

[8] Mohib K, Cherukuri A, Rothstein DM. Regulatory B cells and transplantation: Almost prime time? Current Opinion in Organ Transplantation. 2018;**23**(5):524-532. DOI: 10.1097/MOT.0000000000000559

[9] Schmitz R, Fitch ZW, Schroder PM, Choi AY, Jackson AM, Knechtle SJ, et al. B cells in transplant tolerance and rejection: Friends or foes? Transplant International. 2020;**33**(1):30-40. DOI: 10.1111/tri.13549

[10] Short S, Lewik G, Issa F. An immune atlas of T cells in transplant rejection: Pathways and therapeutic opportunities. Transplantation. 2023;**107**(11):2341-2352. DOI: 10.1097/TP.0000000000004572

[11] Giganti G, Atif M, Mohseni Y, Mastronicola D, Grageda N, Povoleri GA, et al. Treg cell therapy: How cell heterogeneity can make the difference. European Journal of Immunology. 2021;**51**:39-55. DOI: 10.1002/eji.201948131

[12] Grover P, Goel PN, Greene MI. Regulatory T cells: Regulation of identity and function. Frontiers in Immunology. 2021;**12**:750542. DOI: 10.3389/fimmu.2021.750542

[13] Garcia SG, Sandoval-Hellín N, Franquesa M. Regulatory B cell therapy in kidney transplantation. Frontiers in Pharmacology. 2021;**12**:791450. DOI: 10.3389/fphar.2021.791450

[14] Todo S, Yamashita K, Goto R, Zaitsu M, Nagatsu A, Oura T, et al. A pilot study of operational tolerance with regulatory T-cell-based cell therapy in living donor liver transplantation. Hepatology. 2016;**64**:632-643. DOI: 10.1002/hep.28459

[15] Pilat N, Steiner R, Sprent J. Treg therapy for the induction of immune tolerance in transplantation-not lost in translation? International Journal of Molecular Sciences. 2023;**24**(2):1752. DOI: 10.3390/ijms24021752

[16] Sawitzki B, Harden PN, Reinke P, Moreau A, Hutchinson JA, Game DS, et al. Regulatory cell therapy in kidney transplantation (the ONE study): A harmonised design and analysis of seven non-randomised, single-arm, phase 1/2A trials. Lancet. 2020;**395**(10237): 1627-1639. DOI: 10.1016/S0140-6736(20)30167-7. Erratum in: Lancet. 2020 Jun 27;395(10242):1972. doi: 10.1016/S0140-6736(20)31419-7

[17] Leventhal J et al. Tolerance induction in HLA disparate living donor kidney transplantation by donor stem cell infusion: Durable chimerism predicts outcome. Transplantation. 2013;**95**(1):169-176

[18] Hotta K, Hirose T, Kawai T. Clinical trials for renal allograft tolerance induction through combined hematopoietic stem cell transplantation: A narrative review. International Journal of Urology. 2022;**29**:1397-1404

[19] Messner F, Etra JW, Dodd-o JM, Brandacher G, FAST1. Chimerism, transplant tolerance, and beyond. Transplantation. 2019;**103**(8):1556-1567. DOI: 10.1097/TP.0000000000002711

[20] Kawai T, Cosimi AB, Colvin RB, Powelson J, Eason J, Kozlowski T, et al. Mixed allogeneic chimerism and renal allograft tolerance in cynomolgus monkeys. Transplantation. 1995;**59**(2):256-262

[21] El Jurdi N et al. Hematopoietic cell and solid organ transplantation in the same patient: Long-term experience at the University of Minnesota. Transplantation and Cellular Therapy, Official Publication of the American Society for Transplantation and Cellular Therapy; Jan 2021;**27**(1):87.e1-87.e6

[22] Doney KC, Mielcarek M, Stewart FM, Appelbaum FR. Hematopoietic cell transplantation after solid organ transplantation. Biology of Blood and Marrow Transplantation. 2015;**21**(12):2123-2128. DOI: 10.1016/j.bbmt.2015.08.004. Epub 2015 Aug 10

[23] Basak GW, WiktorJedrzejczak W, Labopin M, Schoemans H, Ljungman P, Kobbe G, et al. Allogeneic hematopoietic stem cell transplantation in solid organ transplant recipients: A retrospective, multicenter study of the EBMT. American Journal of Transplantation. 2015;**15**(3):705-714

[24] Shinohara A et al. Hematopoietic stem cell transplantation in solid organ recipients with emphasis on transplant complications: A Nationwide retrospective survey on behalf of the Japan Society for Hematopoietic Stem Cell Transplantation Transplant Complications Working Group. Biology of Blood and Marrow Transplantation. 2020;**26**(1):66-75

[25] Ziliotis M-J, Vauchy C, Deconinck E, Berceanu A, Büchler M, Caillard S, et al. Kidney transplantation after allogeneic hematopoietic. Cell Transplantation. 2024;**9**(4):P1127-P1131. DOI: 10.1016/j.ekir.2024.01.048

[26] Puttarajappa CM, Schinstock CA, Wu CM, Leca N, Kumar V, Vasudev BS, et al. US commentary on the 2020 KDIGO clinical practice guideline on the evaluation and management of candidates for kidney transplantation. American Journal of Kidney Disease. 2021;**77**(6):833-856. DOI: 10.1053/j.ajkd.2020.11.017